T5-CQD-237

Pediatrics

Roslyn Thomas FRCP
Consultant Paediatrician
Northwick Park Hospital
London, UK

David Harvey FRCP DCH
Professor of Paediatrics and Neonatal Medicine
Imperial College School of Medicine
Hammersmith Hospital
London, UK

SECOND EDITION

U.S. EDITOR

Martha Nelson MD
Clinical Instructor Hospital-Perinatal Medicine
Department of Pediatrics
University of Michigan Medical Center
Ann Arbor, Michigan

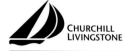

CHURCHILL
LIVINGSTONE

EDINBURGH LONDON NEW YORK PHILADELPHIA SAN FRANCISCO
SYDNEY TORONTO 1998

CHURCHILL LIVINGSTONE
A Division of Harcourt Brace and Company
Limited

© Harcourt Brace and Company Limited 1997

🖉 is a registered trademark of Harcourt Brace
and Company Limited

Adapted from Colour Guide Paediatrics Second
Edition by R. Thomas and D. Harvey 1997

ISBN 0443 05880 6

Library of Congress Cataloging in Publication Data
A catalog record for this book is available from
the Library of Congress.

Medical knowledge is constantly
changing. As new information
becomes available, changes in
treatment, procedures,
equipment, and the use of drugs
become necessary. The authors
and the publishers have, as far as
it is possible, taken care to
ensure that the information given
in this text is accurate and up to
date. However, readers are
strongly advised to confirm that
the information, especially with
regard to drug usage, complies
with current legislation and
standards of practice.

The
publisher's
policy is to use
**paper manufactured
from sustainable forests**

Produced by Longman Asia Limited,
Hong Kong. SWTC/01

For Churchill Livingstone

Publisher: Timothy Horne
Project editor: James Dale
Copy editor: Donna Regen
Project controller: Nancy Arnott
Design direction: Erik Bigland

Contents

Birth to 6 weeks

Gross motor

At birth, there is marked head lag when the infant is pulled from the supine position (Fig. 1). In ventral suspension with the examiner's hand supporting the chest (Fig. 3), the back is rounded and there is some flexion of the hips and knees. By 6 weeks of age, the infant can lift the head when placed in the prone position (Fig. 2) and there is some head control when pulled from supine to sitting.

Fine motor and vision

A baby can see at birth but by 6 weeks can fix vision on objects and will follow horizontally across to 90 degrees.

Hearing and speech

Response to noise will be indicated by startle or quietening to a soothing voice.

Social behavior

The infant will stop crying when picked up to be nursed. Infants also begin to smile in response to familiar noises and faces by 5 weeks.

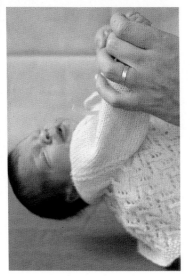

Fig. 1 Head lag.

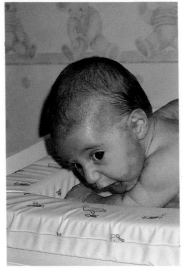

Fig. 2 Lifting head when prone—by 6 weeks.

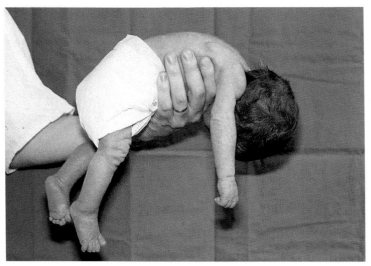

Fig. 3 Ventral suspension showing rounded back.

3–6 months

Gross motor

By 6 months, the infant in the prone position kicks well, pushes up from the forearms, lifting the head and chest (Fig. 4), and begins to roll from front to back. Infants can sit with support or leaning forward into the tripod position (Fig. 5). The age of first sitting alone ranges from $4\frac{1}{2}$ to $8\frac{1}{2}$ months. They begin to weight-bear and to rise to the standing position when supported by the arms or chest.

Fine motor and vision

The infant will reach out for objects with a coarse palmar approach and will clasp and retain small objects placed in the hand. Infants place objects into the mouth and also begin to release objects.

Hearing and speech

The infant can laugh, gurgle, and coo. At about 6 months, they usually begin to babble. Infants will turn when their name is called.

Social behavior

The infant holds on to a bottle or feeding cup when fed and frolics when played with. Infants examine and play with their own hands and place their feet into their mouths (Fig. 6).

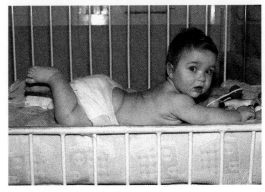

Fig. 4 A press-up at 6 months.

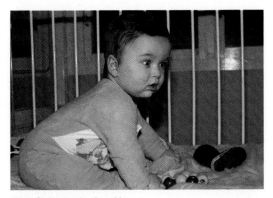

Fig. 5 Sitting in tripod position.

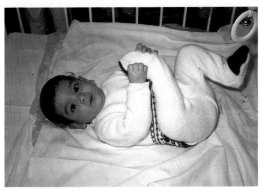

Fig. 6 Playing with feet.

6–9 months

Gross motor	By 6 months, an infant can roll from front to back. Infants sit unsupported with a straight back (Fig. 7). They begin to pivot around on their arms and legs into the crawling position (Fig. 9). They may also begin to crawl on hands and knees.
Fine motor and vision	Small objects are picked up between index finger and thumb in a pincer grasp. Objects are transferred from one hand to the other (Fig. 8).
Hearing and speech	By 9 months, infants shout to gain attention and vocalize nonspecific syllables such as "dada" and "mama".
Social behavior	The baby turns when being talked to and resists when objects are taken from them. Infants try to reach objects out of their reach. They like to feed themselves with their fingers.

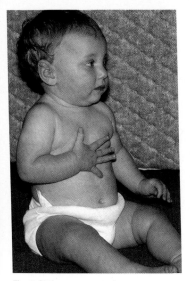

Fig. 7 Sitting unsupported.

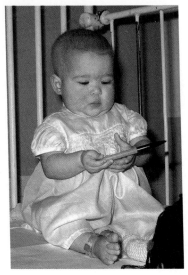

Fig. 8 Transferring objects.

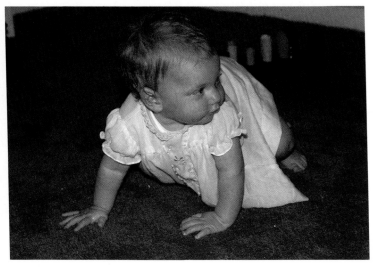

Fig. 9 Getting into a crawling position.

9–12 months

Gross motor

Most infants are crawling by 9–10 months of age. About 10% of normal infants never crawl but move around by rolling, paddling, or bottom shuffling (Fig. 10). Such children are often late walkers, and other family members may have also exhibited this normal variant of motor development. These children may not walk alone until 2 years of age. Children of 9–12 months begin to pull themselves to standing (Fig. 11) and to cruise around the room holding on to furniture.

Fine motor and vision

The infant will bang two cubes together. Infants also look for fallen objects.

Hearing and speech

By 9–12 months, infants usually have one or two recognizable single words in addition to "mama" and "dada".

Social behavior

Infants enjoy imitative games such as clapping hands and waving goodbye but are shy with strangers until the end of the first year.

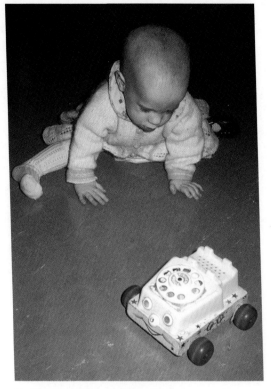

Fig. 10 Normal variant of getting around.

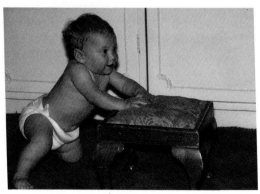

Fig. 11 Getting up to standing.

12–18 months

Gross motor

By 12 months, a child can usually walk with hands held (Fig. 12) and begins to stand alone. Only 3% have not begun to walk by 18 months of age. At that time, the child will be climbing onto chairs and up stairs and will also hold on to toys while walking.

Fine motor and vision

The pincer grip becomes more refined, and tiny objects can be picked up delicately (Fig. 13). The child also points at objects with the index finger (Fig. 14) and casts objects down repeatedly and can be persuaded to give objects to another person on request. The child builds a tower with two or three bricks.

Hearing and speech

There is a vocabulary of several words, and the child usually also repeats their own name. Comprehension is more advanced than speech at this age. The child enjoys looking at pictures in a book and often points and babbles while doing this.

Social behavior

By 12 months, children indicate their wants, usually by pointing. They drink from a cup and help to feed themselves. They also begin to help with dressing. The child learns to throw and enjoys simple games such as peek-a-boo (Fig. 15).

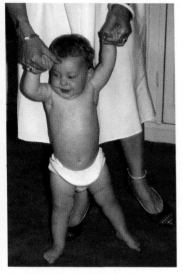

Fig. 12 Walking with help.

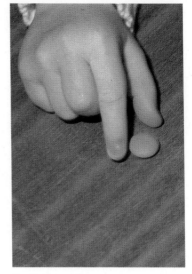

Fig. 13 Pincer grip.

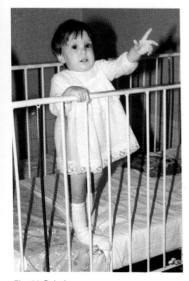

Fig. 14 Pointing.

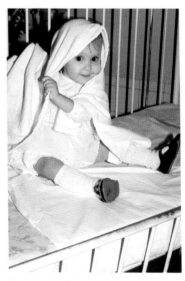

Fig. 15 Peek-a-boo.

2 / Nutrition and growth

Normal growth

Growth in childhood is influenced by genetic, nutritional, and emotional factors as well as specific diseases and hormonal deficiencies. Accurate measurements of height (Figs. 16 and 18), weight, and head circumference should be plotted on centile charts throughout childhood.

Height and weight

Growth in infancy is rapid. This is followed by slow, steady growth in middle childhood until the adolescent growth spurt, after which final adult height is reached and epiphyseal fusion takes place. The growth of most children follows a course similar to those of the centile charts. Height below the third centile occurs in 3% of normal healthy children, and their parents' height should also be measured to assess whether such children have genetic short stature or a disorder of growth. Most preterm and small-for-gestational-age infants achieve normal adult size, unless there is very severe intrauterine growth retardation.

Head growth

The major postnatal growth in brain and head circumference occurs in the first 3 years of life. Asymmetry of the skull (plagiocephaly) and face (Fig. 17) caused by intrauterine posture is common in infancy and usually improves with age. Premature fusion of the skull sutures (craniosynostosis) occasionally results in asymmetry of the skull.

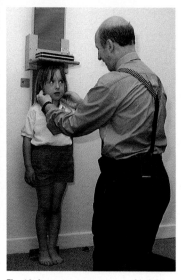

Fig. 16 Accurate measurement of height.

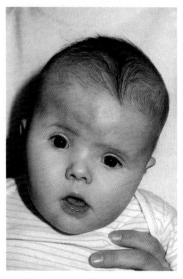

Fig. 17 Asymmetry of face and skull.

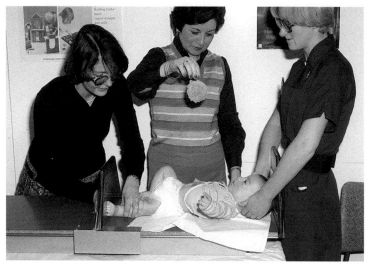

Fig. 18 Measurement of length.

Short stature

Most short children are normal and have short parents. Others may have chromosomal abnormalities such as Turner syndrome, primary or secondary hypopituitarism, hypothyroidism, isolated growth hormone deficiency, chondrodysplasia, or iatrogenic causes (particularly long-term corticosteroid therapy).

Physical examination usually reveals other dysmorphic features in chromosomal abnormalities and chondrodysplasias. In chondrodysplasia, there are usually disproportionately short limbs or trunk (Fig. 19), and skeletal radiographs are abnormal. Juvenile hypothyroidism results in progressive growth failure (Fig. 20), severe retardation of bone age, coarse facies (Fig. 21), and intellectual retardation. In isolated growth hormone deficiency, the child is usually overweight for its height. Serial height measurements show reduced growth velocity, and stimulation tests of pituitary function demonstrate specific failure of growth hormone production. Multiple pituitary hormone failure is usually secondary to neoplasia (particularly craniopharyngioma), radiotherapy, or trauma.

Depends on underlying cause. If a hormonal deficiency is found, specific replacement therapy is indicated. Catch-up growth and height depend on the age at diagnosis and the duration and severity of the underlying disorder.

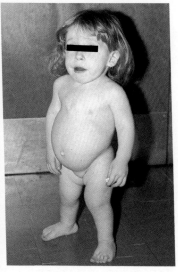

Fig. 19 Short-limbed chondrodysplasia. (By courtesy of Dr. G. Supramanian.)

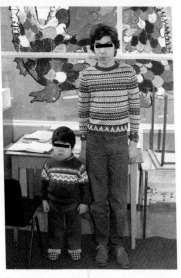

Fig. 20 16-year-old boy with short stature due to hypothyroidism with a normal 16-year-old boy.

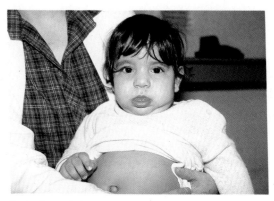

Fig. 21 Coarse facies in juvenile hypothyroidism.

Failure to thrive

Definition

Failure to gain weight at the normal rate in early childhood. Birth weight is normal, but normal weight gain does not occur. If the underlying cause of the problem is not resolved for some time, height and head circumference may also be affected.

Etiology

The most common cause is inadequate dietary intake. Congenital malformations, chromosomal disorders, and specific syndromes can usually be diagnosed or suspected on routine physical examination. The most common causes of malabsorption in childhood are cystic fibrosis and celiac disease.

Clinical features

The weight chart will show progressive deviation from the normal. The buttocks are thin and wasted (Fig. 22), and there is loss of subcutaneous fat with poor muscle bulk (Fig. 23). If failure to thrive is caused by malabsorption, abdominal distension (Fig. 24) is common, and rickets occasionally occurs.

Investigation

Dietary intake must be assessed. Anemia and steatorrhea are suggestive of malabsorption. Sweat test and jejunal biopsy will confirm the diagnoses of cystic fibrosis and celiac disease, respectively.

Obesity

Etiology

This is a common health problem in Western society. It is rarely caused by endocrine disturbance and often has a genetic component.

Clinical features

Weight is greater than expected from height centile even though the child is often quite tall. Skin-fold thickness is excessive.

Management

Prevention or early change in dietary habit is desirable, as established obesity is very difficult to treat.

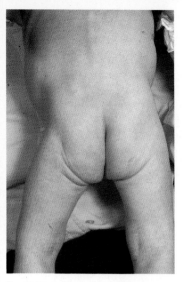

Fig. 22 Wasted buttocks in celiac disease.

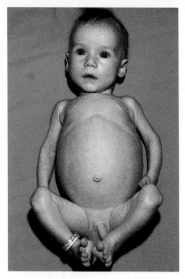

Fig. 23 Failure to thrive with distended abdomen and wasted limbs.

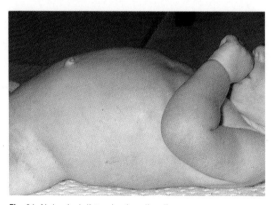

Fig. 24 Abdominal distension in celiac disease.

Malnutrition

Marasmus

Clinical features

Severe generalized undernutrition. In developing countries, it is usually due to failure to breast-feed and inadequate dietary intake. It sometimes occurs in chronic illness. Extreme emaciation (Fig. 25) and increased susceptibility to gastroenteritis and infection are common.

Protein energy malnutrition (PEM or kwashiorkor)

Inadequate dietary protein intake results in edema (Fig. 26), cheilosis (Fig. 27), depigmented and scaly skin, and sparse friable reddish hair (Fig. 28). The infant usually has a poor appetite and is listless and irritable. Fatty infiltration of the liver causes hepatomegaly.

Prevention

Community health education should aim to prevent nutritional deficiency states. Breast-feeding should be encouraged, particularly in developing countries where formula milks are often expensive. Cheap nutritious local foods should be introduced into the infant's diet from 4 to 6 months of age.

Management

Early recognition of deficiency states and gradual reintroduction of an adequate local diet. Associated infections may require treatment, and vitamin supplementation is usually necessary.

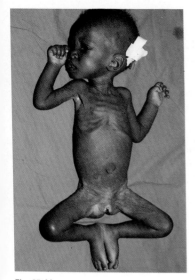

Fig. 25 Marasmus.

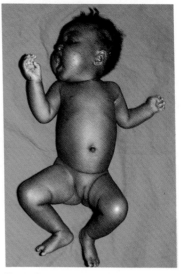

Fig. 26 Protein energy malnutrition (PEM or kwashiorkor).

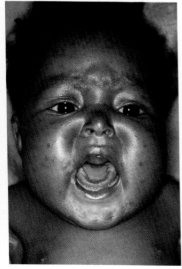

Fig. 27 Cheilosis and depigmented skin in PEM.

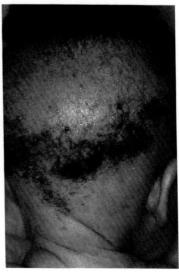

Fig. 28 Sparse friable hair in PEM.

Rickets

Etiology

The most common cause is vitamin D deficiency due to inadequate dietary intake. Malabsorption, liver disease, renal failure, renal tubular dysfunction, and long-term anticonvulsant therapy may also cause rickets.

Clinical features

Swelling of long bone metaphyses, particularly at the wrist (Fig. 29), bowing of the legs, chest deformity, and rachitic rosary (Fig. 30). Craniotabes and delayed closure of the fontanelle may occur in young infants. The child is often irritable and fretful and has bone tenderness and muscle weakness.

Diagnosis

The classic biochemical disturbance is hypocalcemia, hypophosphatemia, and vitamin D deficiency accompanied by a raised bone alkaline phosphatase level. Radiologic signs of rickets include splaying of the metaphyses of long bones with delayed ossification of the epiphyses. Pathologic fractures and deformity of weight-bearing long bones sometimes occur.

Management

Vitamin D supplementation and improved dietary intake. High dosage may be necessary in renal rickets or hereditary hypophosphatemic rickets.

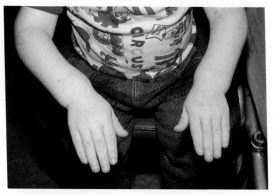

Fig. 29 Swelling of metaphyses at wrists.

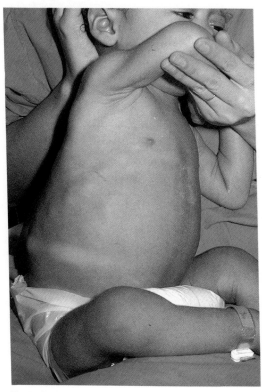

Fig. 30 Rachitic rosary.

Adrenogenital syndrome

Synonyms

Congenital adrenal hyperplasia.

Incidence

1 in 5,000 live births.

Etiology

Autosomal recessive disorder due to enzyme deficiency in cortisol and aldosterone synthesis resulting in excessive testosterone production. The most common type is due to 21-hydroxylase deficiency. Prenatal diagnosis is possible.

Clinical features

Affected females are virilized from birth (Fig. 31) and may be confused for males with severe hypospadias and bilateral cryptorchidism. If virilization is not recognized early, particularly in male infants, they may collapse in the second week of life with a life-threatening adrenal crisis.

Diagnosis

Elevated plasma 17-hydroxyprogesterone level, plasma ACTH, and urinary steroid excretion.

Management

Salt-losing crises require urgent resuscitation with intravenous saline. Replacement hydrocortisone and a salt-retaining steroid, fludrocortisone, are required for long-term suppression of the hyperplastic adrenal glands.

Cushing syndrome

Etiology

Excessive cortisol production usually due to bilateral adrenal hyperplasia caused by pituitary adenomata. It is occasionally caused by local adrenal adenoma or carcinoma. High-dosage administration of corticosteroids will produce similar clinical features.

Clinical features

Moon facies (Fig. 32), truncal obesity, hirsutism, acne, striae (Fig. 33), growth retardation, osteoporosis, and muscle wasting.

Management

Surgery with or without radiotherapy.

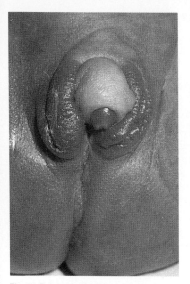

Fig. 31 Enlarged clitoris in congenital adrenal hyperplasia.

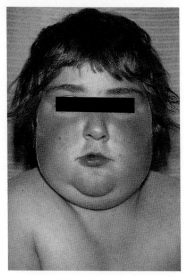

Fig. 32 Moon facies in Cushing syndrome.

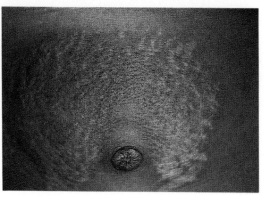

Fig. 33 Abdominal striae in Cushing syndrome.

Precocious puberty

Definition

Development of secondary sex characteristics before the age of 8 years in girls and 10 years in boys.

Incidence

Early puberty is more common in girls than boys, and isolated premature thelarche (breast development) (Fig. 34) is relatively common.

Etiology

In physiologic early puberty, there is premature activation of the hypothalamo-pituitary-gonadal axis. Cerebral tumors, particularly pineal tumors in boys, gonadal or adrenal tumors, and exogenous steroid administration also cause early development of secondary sex characteristics.

Clinical features and diagnosis

Careful physical examination may help to distinguish between physiologic but early onset of puberty and pathologic development (Figs. 35 and 36). Discrepancies from the usual sequence of pubertal development, such as pubic hair but no breast development, are unlikely to be physiologic. Abdominal palpation and ultrasound are important in the detection of adrenal or gonadal tumors. Intracranial tumors must always be excluded.

Management

Pathologic causes such as hypothyroidism or tumors require specific treatment. Short stature is the major long-term physical disadvantage of early puberty because of the shorter period of prepubertal growth before epiphyseal fusion. Early puberty is also psychologically upsetting to both child and parents. Drug therapy may be used to suppress gonadotropin release until the child reaches an appropriate age.

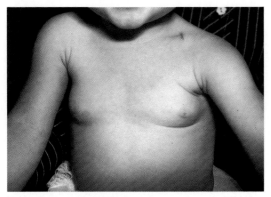

Fig. 34 Premature breast development.

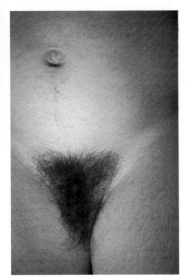

Fig. 35 Sexual precocity at 5 years of age (adrenal tumor).

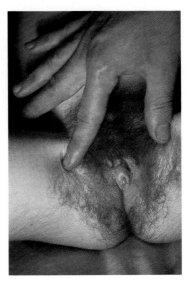

Fig. 36 Pathologic enlargement of clitoris.

Hypothyroidism

Incidence

Relatively common; congenital hypothyroidism occurs in 1 in 4,000 live births.

Etiology

Congenital hypothyroidism is usually due to thyroid agenesis. It is occasionally due to inherited dysgenesis of hormone synthesis.

Clinical features

Coarse facies (Fig. 37), dry skin, hoarse voice and cry, and paucity of spontaneous activity. Hypothermia, hypotonia, and poor weight gain are common. Umbilical hernia, constipation, and prolonged jaundice sometimes occur in neonates. Intellectual retardation is the major long-term effect in young infants. Some have cerebellar ataxia, myopia, and squints. In juvenile hypothyroidism occurring in later childhood, there is growth failure but very little intellectual impairment if thyroid function has been normal during the early critical period of brain growth.

Management

Replacement therapy (Fig. 38) with L-thyroxine for life. Dosage is adjusted to achieve normal growth and bone age as well as suppression of thyroid-stimulating hormone.

Hyperthyroidism

Incidence

Uncommon. Neonatal thyrotoxicosis may occur in infants of mothers with a history of thyrotoxicosis and thyroid-stimulating immunoglobulins.

Clinical features

Young infants have tachycardia, vomiting, sweating, poor weight gain, and irritability. Older children may also have rapid growth, tremor, and proptosis and goiter (Fig. 39).

Management

Antithyroid drugs such as carbimazole until spontaneous remission, usually within 2 years. Some require thyroidectomy. Neonatal thyrotoxicosis resolves within a few weeks; sometimes no treatment is needed.

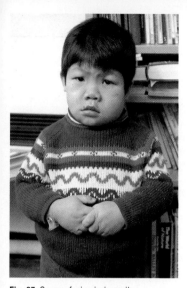

Fig. 37 Coarse facies in juvenile hypothyroidism.

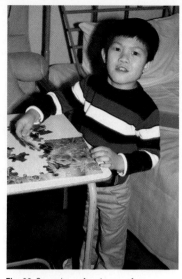

Fig. 38 Same boy after 1 year of replacement therapy.

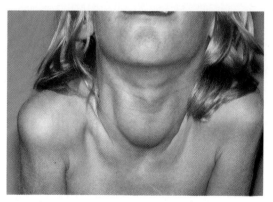

Fig. 39 Goiter in hyperthyroidism.

Measles

Clinical features

After an incubation period of 10–14 days, there is a prodromal illness with fever, coryza, conjunctivitis, and cough. The child is extremely miserable, and for about 24 h before and after the rash appears, tiny white spots on a bright red background (Koplik's spots) may be seen on the buccal mucosa of the cheek. After 3–4 days, a florid, maculopapular rash appears on the face and behind the ears (Fig. 40). The rash becomes more confluent as it spreads down the trunk (Fig. 41); bronzing and desquamation occur after 4–7 days.

Complications

Bronchopneumonia and otitis media are common; encephalitis occurs in 1 in 1,000 children with measles. Rarely, a slowly progressive neurodegenerative disorder (subacute sclerosing panencephalitis) occurs some years after acute measles.

Immunization

Measles carries a high morbidity; mortality is high in children with malnutrition or immunodeficiency. Immunization in a triple vaccine with mumps and rubella (MMR) is given at 12–15 months of age. Many states in the United States recommend a booster at 12 years of age.

German measles (rubella)

Clinical features

The incubation period is 14–21 days. There is mild illness with transient, nonspecific pink macular rash lasting only a few days. Generalized lymphadenopathy, particularly with involvement of the suboccipital nodes, is common.

Complications

Thrombocytopenia occasionally occurs. Arthritis is more common in adolescent girls. Rubella embryopathy affecting the developing fetus in the first trimester of pregnancy is the most devastating complication.

Immunization

MMR vaccine is given routinely at 1 year of age. All girls who have not had MMR should be vaccinated before puberty.

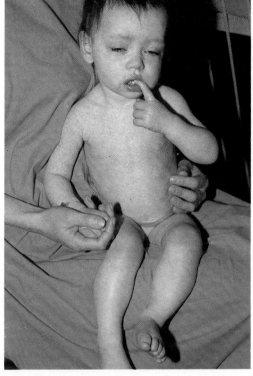

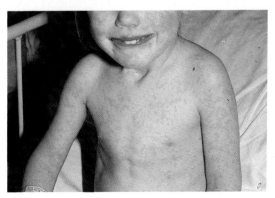

Fig. 40 Miserable child with measles.

Fig. 41 Measles rash.

Mumps

Clinical features

Fever and enlargement of one or both parotid glands (Fig. 42) occur 14–21 days after contact by a susceptible individual. Many children have subclinical infection. The brawny, swollen glands are painful and tender and often accompanied by earache or trismus. Submandibular salivary glands may also be affected, and differentiation from lymphadenopathy may occasionally be difficult.

Complications

Meningitis is common but mild. It may precede or occur in the absence of parotid swelling. Pancreatitis and epididymo-orchitis occur more often in adults.

Immunization

Vaccination is now given routinely as a part of MMR at 1 year of age.

Infectious mononucleosis (glandular fever)

Clinical features

Sporadic infection caused by the Epstein–Barr virus after an incubation period of 4–14 days. Anorexia, malaise, fever, and generalized lymphadenopathy are prominent symptoms. There may be petechiae on the palate, and in children a severe exudative tonsillitis often occurs. A macular rash occurs in approximately 20% of cases, and in 90% if ampicillin is given (Fig. 43).

Diagnosis

Atypical mononuclear cells appear in the blood film, and agglutination tests (such as Paul–Bunnell test) may be positive in the early weeks.

Complications

Hepatitis is common. Nonspecific symptoms of fever and malaise may persist for several weeks or occasionally months.

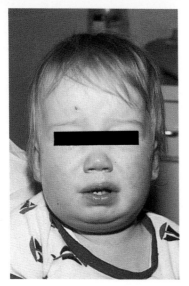

Fig. 42 Parotid swelling in mumps.

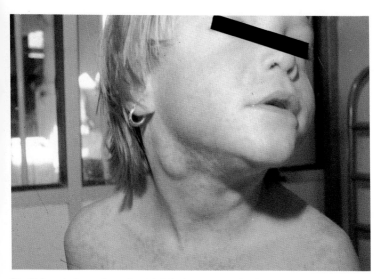

Fig. 43 Lymphadenopathy and rash in infectious mononucleosis.

Herpes zoster

Chickenpox (varicella)

Clinical features

Incubation period 14–21 days. The spots occur in crops that rapidly progress from macules to papules to vesicles (Fig. 44). The vesicle becomes crusted, and the child remains infectious until the scales separate 10–14 days later, often leaving pitted scars.

Complications

Chickenpox is usually a mild illness, except when the child is immunodeficient. Encephalitis is rare, but when it occurs, the predominant sign is ataxia with onset several weeks after the acute illness. Hemorrhagic chickenpox (Fig. 45) is a very uncommon but severe form of the illness.

Shingles (herpes zoster)

Uncommon in children. Vesicles have the typical dermatome distribution (Fig. 46). Itching is a common symptom, but postherpetic neuralgia is uncommon in children.

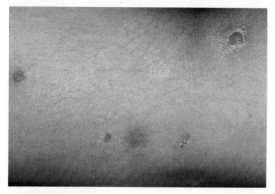

Fig. 44 Chickenpox.

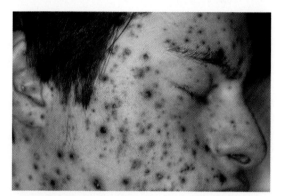

Fig. 45 Hemorrhagic chickenpox.

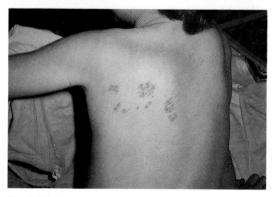

Fig. 46 Shingles.

Herpes simplex

Clinical features

Primary herpes simplex infection may produce a severe gingivostomatitis in young children. Multiple painful blisters or ulcers occur around the mouth, on the lips (Figs. 47 and 49), and on buccal mucous membranes. The child is usually extremely miserable, with excessive dribbling and salivation, fever, irritability, and difficulty in swallowing. Recurrent herpes simplex causes the simple common cold sore.

Complications

Dehydration may occur when there is inadequate fluid intake because of the painful mouth and difficulty in swallowing. Herpes encephalitis is a rare but serious complication with high mortality and morbidity.

Management

Sympathetic nursing, analgesia, and adequate fluid intake are necessary. The primary infection is usually self-limiting within 2 weeks. Early infection within 48 h of onset may respond to topical acyclovir. Acyclovir is also used for systemic complications.

Hemophilus cellulitis

Clinical features

Hemophilus influenzae may cause severe cellulitis affecting the face, particularly the cheek, periorbital region, and neck (Fig. 48).

Management

The condition responds to an appropriate antibiotic—usually ampicillin, chloramphenicol, or a cephalosporin.

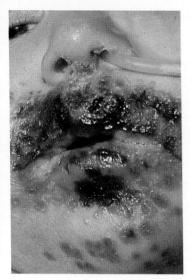

Fig. 47 Herpes stomatitis.

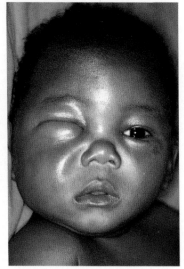

Fig. 48 Hemophilus cellulitis of the face.

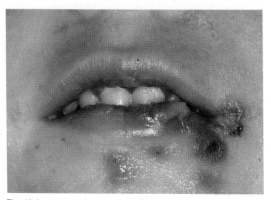

Fig. 49 Less severe herpes stomatitis.

Staphylococcal infection

Clinical features

Impetigo, the most common superficial staphylococcal infection, is highly contagious. Individual lesions begin as erythematous spots that rapidly increase in size and develop brown crusts (Fig. 50). Group A β-hemolytic strep is often the inciting pathogen in impetigo in many parts of the United States.

Toxic epidermal necrolysis (scalded skin syndrome) is caused by toxins of staphylococcal phage types 71 or 22. Initially, there is intense redness and pain, resembling a superficial scald. Minimal trauma may result in a positive Nikolsky's sign (separation of epidermis from dermis because of edema between the two layers of skin). Generalized exfoliation of the skin often occurs.

Management

A systemic antistaphylococcal antibiotic such as flucloxacillin is given. Tetracycline should never be used in children because of the risk of staining the teeth (Fig. 51). General hygiene such as frequent handwashing and short clean finger nails will help to limit cross-infection. Nasal carriage of staphylococci in the internal nares will be reduced by the use of antiseptic cream or oral rifampicin for recurrent sepsis. Treatment of staph infections frequently involves the use of Nafcillin or oral Augmentin in the United States.

Osteomyelitis

Clinical features

About 90% of cases are caused by *Staphylococcus aureus*. The metaphyses of the long bones are usually affected. There are local signs of acute inflammation and exquisite bony tenderness. Fever and toxemia often occur.

Diagnosis and management

Blood cultures usually identify the organism. Radioisotope bone scan may reveal a "hot spot" earlier than radiographs, which rarely show any abnormality before the second week. Surgical drainage is sometimes necessary. Systemic antibiotics are given for several months. With adequate treatment, chronic osteomyelitis (Fig. 52) is now rare.

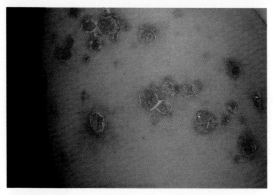

Fig. 50 Impetigo.

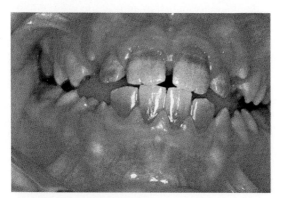

Fig. 51 Tetracycline staining of teeth.

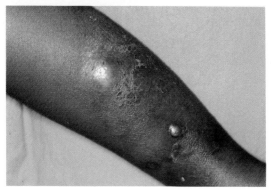

Fig. 52 Chronic osteomyelitis.

Meningitis

Etiology

The most common organisms causing bacterial meningitis in children younger than the age of 5 years are *Hemophilus influenzae*, meningococci, or pneumococci.

Clinical features

Specific signs such as headache and neck stiffness occur in older children but are often absent in young infants. Infants often present with non-specific signs of irritability, drowsiness, vomiting, anorexia, convulsions, or fever. Bulging fontanelle, high-pitched cry, and arching of the back (opisthotonos) (Fig. 53) are late signs.

Diagnosis

High index of suspicion in any ill child with unexplained fever or convulsions. Cerebrospinal fluid examination and culture will confirm the diagnosis.

Management

Broad-spectrum antibiotics until the specific organism and sensitivities are known. Contacts to those with meningococcal infection (particularly meningitis) should receive antibiotic prophylaxis (e.g., Rifampin).

Meningococcemia

Clinical features

An acute fulminating septicemia with shock and a purpuric rash (Fig. 54). Meningococcal septicemia has a high mortality.

Diagnosis

Blood cultures should be taken. Antigen testing is very useful, particularly when antibodies have already been given. Lumbar puncture should be considered but may be contraindicated in a very ill child.

Management

High-dosage penicillin and treatment for vascular collapse. Penicillin should be given at once to any child with a suspicious rash.

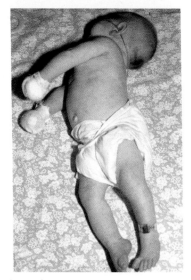

Fig. 53 Opisthotonos.

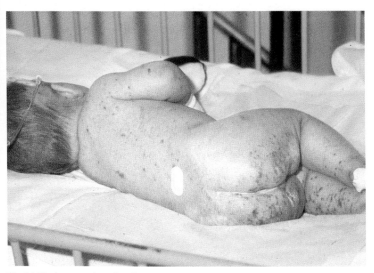

Fig. 54 Meningococcal septicemia.

Erysipelas

Etiology   Streptococcal skin infection.

Clinical features   Spreading cellulitis with a well-defined edge (Fig. 55). A red flare is sometimes seen spreading along the lymphatic drainage.

Management   High-dosage penicillin.

Tuberculosis

Etiology   *Mycobacterium tuberculosis.* Primary infection may present in the lung or as enlarged lymph nodes. It is contracted by droplet spread, usually from asymptomatic adults.

Clinical features   Primary tuberculosis is usually asymptomatic. Hematogenous spread and meningitis are most common in the very young and in children with malnutrition or intercurrent infection. Pulmonary tuberculosis with chronic cough occurs in later life.

Diagnosis   Sensitivity to tuberculin as shown by a positive Mantoux reaction (Fig. 56) develops within 4–8 weeks after infection. Chest radiograph may show hilar lymphadenopathy or a segmental lesion.

Management   Combination chemotherapy with isoniazid and rifampicin for 6–12 months, and occasionally other drugs, particularly for miliary spread or tuberculosis meningitis.

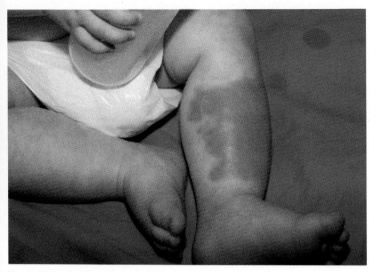

Fig. 55 Well-defined erythema (erysipelas).

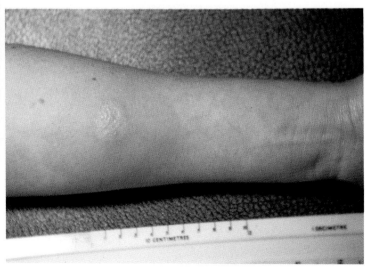

Fig. 56 Positive Mantoux reaction.

Eczema

Incidence

Common; affects 3% of children. Onset usually within first 2 years of life.

Inheritance

Often family history of other atopic disorders (e.g., asthma, hay fever, allergy).

Clinical features

Itchy plaques with excoriation and lichenification (Fig. 57), characteristically occurring on the face, behind the knees, antecubital fossae, and wrists, but can occur anywhere (Fig. 58). The skin is often dry, and itching is a prominent symptom. Secondary infection is common because of scratching.

Investigation

Eosinophilia, raised serum IgE, or positive skin tests are sometimes helpful in the general diagnosis of atopy but are rarely useful in clinical management, as multiple factors are usually involved.

Management

Soap should be avoided, and emollient oil or emulsifying ointment used instead. Aqueous cream can be used liberally on the dry skin. Weak corticosteroid cream may be applied sparingly to bad patches during acute flareups. Systemic antihistamines are sometimes useful to control itching and scratching, which occur particularly during sleep. When there is a clear history of aggravation by certain foods, an exclusion diet may help.

Course and prognosis

Fluctuating course, usually with improvement in later childhood.

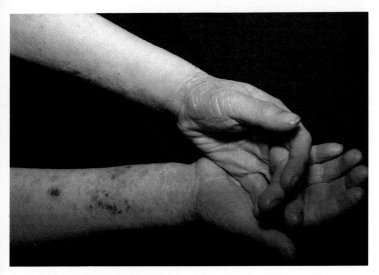

Fig. 57 Typical eczematous rash on arms.

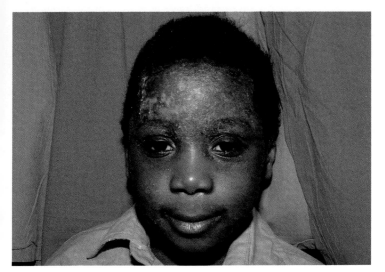

Fig. 58 Eczema on face.

Diaper rash

Etiology

Usually due to irritation from prolonged wearing of wet diapers—sometimes called "ammonical dermatitis". Monilial infection and seborrheic dermatitis are the other main rashes in the diaper area.

Clinical features

Erythema, umbilicated pustules, and ulceration of the perineum and sometimes the genitalia (Fig. 59), but usually sparing the groin flexures. The presence of discrete satellite lesions or involvement of the flexures is suggestive of monilial infection (Fig. 60). In babies with loose stools, there is often perianal erythema.

Management

Diapers should be changed frequently. In simple diaper rash, exposure of the perineum and a protective barrier cream is all that is required. Monilial infection responds to topical nystatin or miconazole cream. *Monilia* should always be considered when a rash does not respond to simple treatment. Seborrheic dermatitis often requires the application of a weak steroid cream.

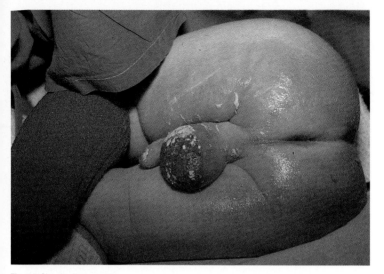

Fig. 59 Simple diaper rash.

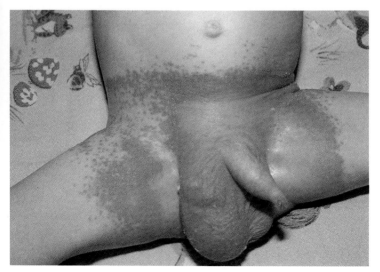

Fig. 60 Monilial infection with discrete satellite lesions.

Seborrheic dermatitis

Etiology
Very common in young infants; etiology unknown.

Clinical features
Distinctive greasy, scaly, erythematous rash or plaques (Fig. 61), which usually appear within the first few months of life. The eyebrows, skin behind the ears, and perineum are commonly affected. Thick greasy scales are often found on the scalp, where the condition is commonly called "cradle cap" (Fig. 62). Occasionally, there may be discoid lesions on the trunk spreading up from a diaper rash (diaper psoriasis) (Fig. 63). In mild forms, seborrheic dermatitis may be mistakenly diagnosed as atopic eczema, particularly when the rash affects the flexures. There is never any systemic illness, even with widespread seborrheic dermatitis (Leiner syndrome), but secondary infection sometimes occurs.

Management
Mild corticosteroid cream such as 1% hydrocortisone. Cradle cap usually responds to a keratolytic shampoo or cream but often recurs.

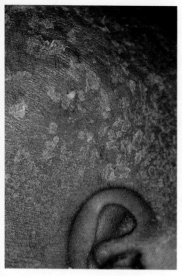

Fig. 61 Typical seborrheic plaques.

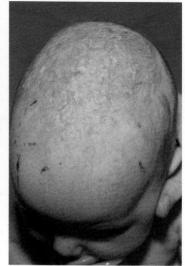

Fig. 62 Cradle cap.

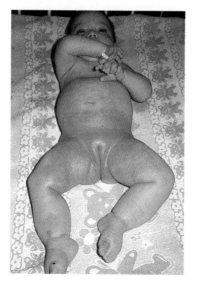

Fig. 63 Diaper psoriasis.

Urticaria

Etiology

A common allergic manifestation, but the offending allergen is often not identified. Some recurrent cases are caused by sensitivity to food-coloring agents.

Clinical features

Intensely itchy, erythematous rash with wheals. The pattern of the rash is constantly changing and may leave areas of bruising when the wheals subside. There is often marked edema, particularly around the eyes and mouth, where it is called "angioneurotic edema" (Fig. 64).

Management

Acute respiratory obstruction caused by severe swelling of the mouth and tongue may be life-threatening; it responds to subcutaneous adrenaline. Systemic antihistamines may be helpful in urticaria. Food exclusion diets may help some children with recurrent urticaria. Some cases of chronic or recurrent urticaria are due to familial acetylcholinesterase deficiency.

Erythema multiforme and Stevens–Johnson syndrome

Etiology

Idiosyncratic reactions, often to drugs such as penicillin or sulfonamides.

Clinical features

Erythema multiforme shows widespread target lesions (Fig. 65). Stevens–Johnson is a more severe illness; it begins as a bullous eruption that rapidly progresses to widespread skin loss (Fig. 66). There is always involvement of the mucous membranes of the mouth, rectum, vagina, or conjunctiva.

Management

Discontinue the offending drug. Barrier nursing, strict fluid and electrolyte balance, and prevention of infection are important. In severe cases, mortality is high, particularly if septicemia occurs.

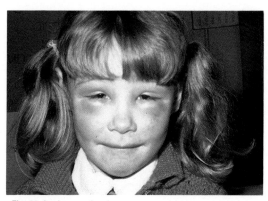

Fig. 64 Angioneurotic edema.

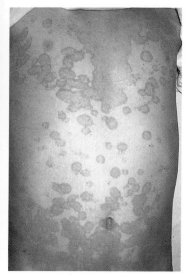

Fig. 65 Target lesions of erythema multiforme.

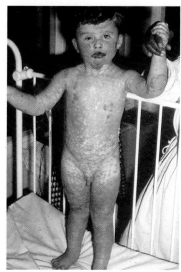

Fig. 66 Stevens–Johnson syndrome.

Henoch–Schönlein purpura

Synonym	Anaphylactoid purpura.
Incidence	Common; often occurs in small epidemics.
Etiology	Diffuse vasculitis of unknown etiology; there is often a history of a recent viral upper respiratory tract infection.
Clinical features	The pathognomonic feature is a purpuric rash on the buttocks, extensor surfaces of the legs and arms (Figs. 67–69), and sometimes the face. The lesions are often papular and bullae are sometimes present. Localized edema of the face, hands, feet, and scrotum often accompany the typical rash, and flitting arthritis affecting the large peripheral joints is common. Colicky abdominal pain is a troublesome symptom and hematemesis, melena or intussusception occur in a few cases. Hematuria occurs in approximately 70% of children with Henoch–Schönlein purpura, but progressive renal disease occurs in less than 1%.
Management	Other causes of purpura should always be excluded. Treatment is symptomatic, and analgesia and bed rest are usually all that is required. Corticosteroids may be indicated if there are severe gastrointestinal symptoms or progressive renal involvement.
Course and prognosis	The majority resolve rapidly, although further episodes or recurrences are common in the first few weeks. The prognosis is more serious if acute nephritis or nephrotic syndrome is present.

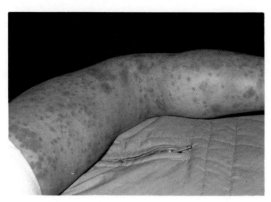

Fig. 67 Typical purpura on the leg.

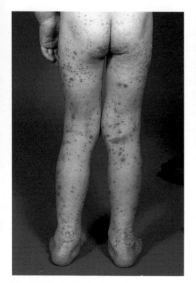

Fig. 68 Classic distribution of
Henoch–Schönlein purpura.

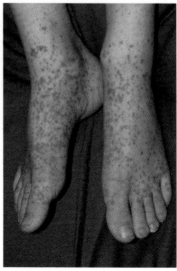

Fig. 69 Purpura on feet.

Erythema nodosum

Incidence	Common, particularly in black children.
Etiology	May be associated with streptococcal infection, tuberculosis, sarcoidosis, *Mycoplasma* infection, drug sensitivity (particularly to sulfonamides), or inflammatory bowel disease. In most cases, no underlying condition will be found.
Clinical features	Exquisitely tender, raised erythematous nodules most frequently occurring over the pretibial region (Fig. 70) but may also occur around the elbows and on the forearms. They often occur in crops over a period of several weeks or occasionally months and may be associated with fever and arthralgia, particularly when the nodules occur over joints. The skin lesions resolve into the same color changes as a bruise.

Dermoid cysts

Etiology	Developmental anomalies that are found along the suture lines of the skull.
Clinical features	Firm, nontender subcutaneous swellings typically found around the orbit or in the midline of the skull anywhere from the occiput to the base of the nose. The most common site is at the lateral margin of the orbit where the dermoid cyst is known as an "external angular dermoid" (Fig. 71).
Course and prognosis	Dermoid cysts usually increase slowly in size. They sometimes become infected.
Management	Surgery to remove the dermoid cyst is usually required for cosmetic reasons or because of recurrent infection.

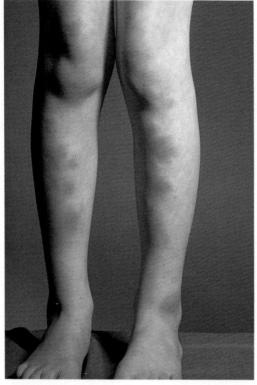

Fig. 70 Erythema nodosum.

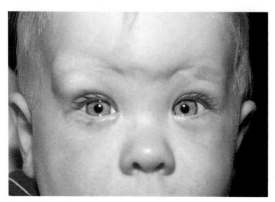

Fig. 71 External angular dermoid.

Fungal infections and infestations

Scabies
Intensely itchy, excoriated, erythematous papular rash (Fig. 72), sometimes with burrows visible to the naked eye. Scabies may occur anywhere on the body but is said to be most common between the fingers and around the wrists. Scabies is spread by close human contact. The whole family should be treated with topical lindane or malathion; clothes and bed linen should be thoroughly washed if recurrence is to be avoided.

Tinea
Tinea (ringworm) causes circular erythematous patches with a scaly center. When tinea affects the scalp, there may be hair loss with circular patches of baldness. Tinea corporis usually responds to topical antifungals such as miconazole. Systemic griseofulvin may be necessary when there is extensive hair or nail involvement.

Monilia
Oral thrush is common in young infants. *Candida* also gives rise to a characteristic diaper rash with erythematous ulcerated satellite lesions. In later childhood, oral thrush may occur when the child is taking corticosteroids or when there is an immunodeficiency syndrome (Fig. 73).

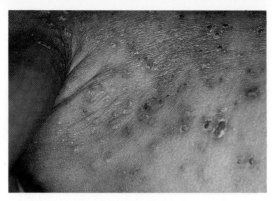

Fig. 72 Scabies infestation with excoriation.

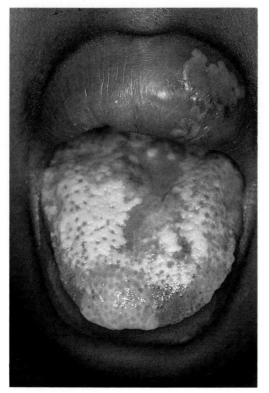

Fig. 73 Oral thrush with severe ulceration.

Psoriasis

Incidence

Uncommon in childhood, and when it occurs there is usually a strong family history.

Etiology

Unknown.

Clinical features

Erythematous, scaly lesions that form plaques (Figs. 74 and 75), typically on the elbows and knees and around the hairline and scalp. When the lesion is scratched lightly, it produces a silvery appearance.

Management and course

The tendency to psoriasis is usually life-long. Treatment depends on the severity of the lesions. Corticosteroids, coal tar, and salicylic acid ointments are the mainstay of treatment.

Cavernous hemangioma

Incidence and etiology

Common congenital malformation of blood vessels usually involving skin or mucous membrane.

Clinical features

Often large blood-filled channels located deeply in the subcutaneous or submucous areas (Fig. 76).

Management

Treatment is only required if there is significant bleeding, thrombocytopenia, or cosmetic embarrassment. Surgical excision is often difficult; sclerosing agents are sometimes used.

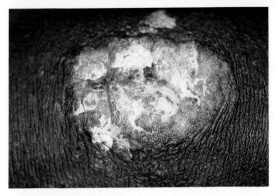

Fig. 74 Severe psoriasis.

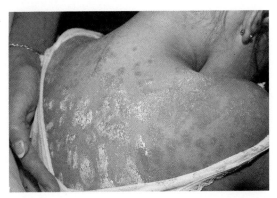

Fig. 75 Multiple plaques of psoriasis.

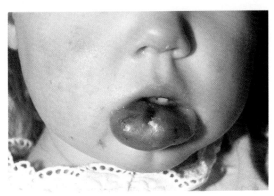

Fig. 76 Cavernous hemangioma of lower lip.

Kawasaki disease

Mucocutaneous lymph node syndrome.

Most common in Japan but reported worldwide.

Prolonged febrile illness with fleeting erythematous rash, sore tongue, cracked lips, and lymphadenopathy. During the second week after the fever has subsided, there is typical peeling of the hands and feet (Fig. 77).

Coronary artery aneurysms associated with thrombocytosis occur in a few children. Salicylates and dipyridamole may prevent the development of coronary artery aneurysms. Intravenous gamma globulin may reduce the cardiac complications.

Keloid

Excessive scar formation (Fig. 78) often after minimal trauma. Common in black population.

Surgical excision is difficult because of the tendency to increasing keloid formation.

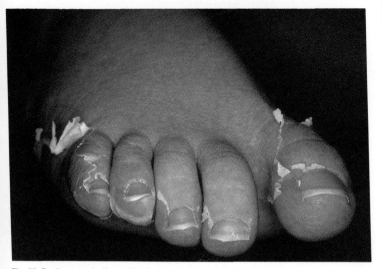

Fig. 77 Peeling toes in Kawasaki disease. (By courtesy of Dr. R. Briggs.)

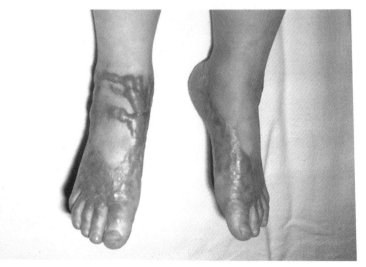

Fig. 78 Keloid after burns.

Alopecia areata

Incidence

Uncommon; alopecia areata totalis is very rare. There is an increased incidence in Down syndrome.

Etiology

Unknown; but sometimes occurs during periods of stress.

Clinical features

Alopecia areata commonly causes localized hair loss on the scalp. It can usually be distinguished from tinea capitis by the characteristic margin of exclamation mark hair shafts and the absence of erythema and scaling (Fig. 79).

Course and prognosis

Usually self-limiting but occasionally may progress to alopecia totalis, which results in total body hair loss. There is no effective treatment.

Pigmented nevi

Clinical features

Discrete brown or black pigmented skin lesions. The lesion is usually not elevated during childhood but may become palpable during adult life. Some congenital pigmented nevi contain hair follicles (Fig. 80). Multiple pigmented nevi are seen in certain syndromes such as neurofibromatosis.

Management

Junctional nevi occasionally develop into malignant melanoma in adults, but this is rare. Most pigmented nevi are harmless (Fig. 81). Surgical excision or dermabrasion may be required for cosmetic reasons.

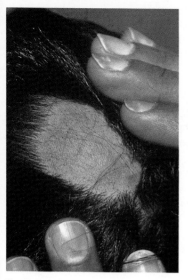

Fig. 79 Scalp hair loss in alopecia areata.

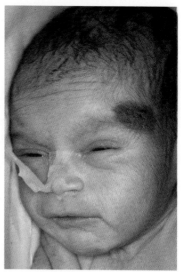

Fig. 80 Congenital pigmented hairy nevus.

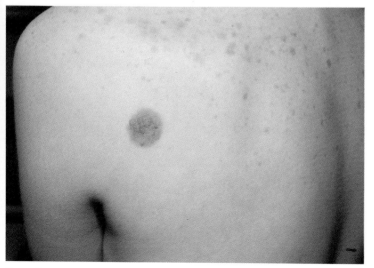

Fig. 81 Multiple pigmented nevi.

6 / Gastrointestinal disorders

Gastroenteritis

Incidence

The most common cause of death in young infants in developing countries where early weaning and malnutrition are common.

Etiology

Rotavirus infection is a common cause of gastroenteritis in infants in winter months. *Escherichia coli*, *Salmonella*, *Shigella*, and *Campylobacter* are the common causes of bacterial gastroenteritis.

Clinical features

Diarrhea, vomiting, and colicky abdominal pain. The most serious complication is dehydration due to excessive water loss or inadequate fluid intake. In mild-to-moderate dehydration (up to 5%), the child is thirsty and lethargic and has sunken eyes and loss of skin turgor (Figs. 82 and 83). In moderate-to-severe dehydration (5–10%), there may be tachycardia and signs of peripheral circulatory collapse. Moderate dehydration often manifests with decreased urine output.

Management

Recognition of dehydration and adequate fluid and electrolyte replacement is important. Frequent administration of an oral glucose electrolyte solution is usually possible, except when there is shock. Intravenous therapy will then be necessary.

Intestinal parasites

Incidence

Common cause of malabsorption, anemia, and chronic diarrhea in developing countries.

Etiology and clinical features

Giardia lamblia is a protozoal infestation that causes acute diarrhea and sometimes chronic malabsorption. *Ascaris lumbricoides* (roundworm) (Fig. 84) causes colicky abdominal pain and gut obstruction. *Ankylostoma* (hookworm) is a common cause of iron deficiency anemia in tropical countries.

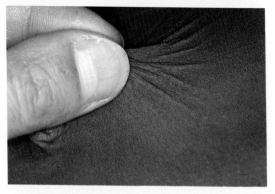

Fig. 82 Dehydration with dry skin.

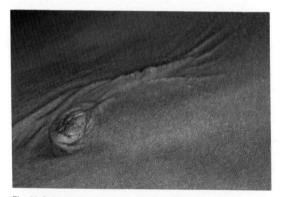

Fig. 83 Dehydration showing poor skin turgor after release.

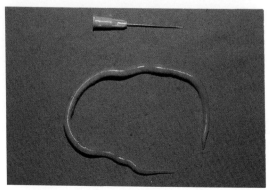

Fig. 84 *Ascaris lumbricoides* (roundworm).

Celiac disease

Synonyms Gluten sensitivity; gluten intolerance.

Etiology Permanent intolerance of dietary wheat, rye, and sometimes barley and oats.

Incidence The world-wide incidence is 1 in 3,000–5,000 live births. The recent impression is that celiac disease is becoming less common.

Clinical features Most children have signs within the first 2 years of life. There may be poor weight gain after introduction of gluten-containing solids, but signs are often more insidious. Vomiting, diarrhea, and abdominal distension are common. Anorexia, irritability with miserable facies (Fig. 85), hypotonia, and wasted buttocks (Figs. 86 and 87) occur. Sometimes failure to thrive or growth failure is the only sign.

Diagnosis Jejunal biopsy, showing total villous atrophy and inflammatory infiltration of the lamina propria, is the definitive investigation.

Management Gluten-free diet. Supplementation with iron and vitamins is often necessary after diagnosis. Lactose or cow's milk protein intolerance sometimes occurs.

Course and prognosis Gastrointestinal symptoms, mood disturbance, and growth failure improve with a gluten-free diet. There is an increased risk of intestinal lymphoma in adult life.

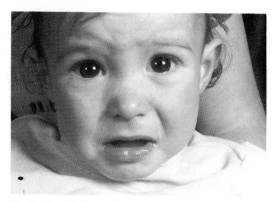

Fig. 85 Miserable facies of celiac child.

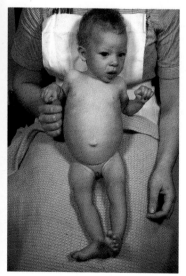

Fig. 86 Abdominal distension.

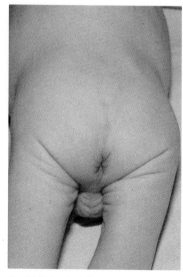

Fig. 87 Abdominal distension and wasted buttocks.

Pyloric stenosis

Etiology

Hypertrophy of the smooth muscle of pylorus of obscure etiology. First-born male infants often affected.

Clinical features

Onset of vomiting within a few weeks of birth. Classically, there is projectile vomiting with failure to thrive and constipation. During feeding, a pyloric mass can usually be palpated, and visible peristalsis may be seen in the upper abdomen (Fig. 88). In difficult cases, an ultrasound examination is helpful.

Management

Surgery (Ramstedt's pyloromyotomy) after rehydration and correction of electrolyte imbalance.

Intussusception

Incidence

Common cause of gut obstruction in infancy.

Clinical features

Sudden onset of colicky abdominal pain, with loose stools often blood-stained (red-currant jelly stools). A sausage-shaped bowel mass may be palpable.

Management

Gentle barium enema (Fig. 89) will confirm the diagnosis and may be curative in cases of recent onset. Surgery may be required for intussusception when the diagnosis is delayed.

Hirschsprung's disease

Etiology

Absence of ganglionic cells in the colon.

Clinical features

May cause acute neonatal intestinal obstruction (Fig. 90) or chronic constipation in older children.

Management

Barium enema and anorectal manometry assist in the diagnosis; rectal biopsy is always necessary for confirmation. Colostomy relieves the acute obstruction; resection of the aganglionic segment and a pull-through anastomosis are performed later.

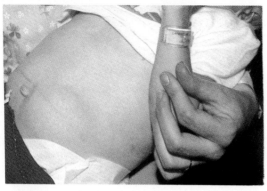

Fig. 88 Visible peristalsis in pyloric stenosis.

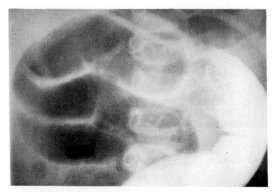

Fig. 89 Intussusception.

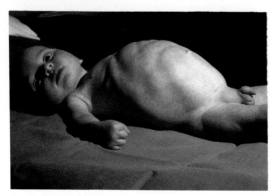

Fig. 90 Distended abdomen in Hirschsprung's disease. (By courtesy of Dr. T. Lissauer.)

Hypospadias

The most common minor abnormality of the male genitalia; occurs in 1 in 350 boys. Malposition of the urethral orifice varies in severity from perineal (Fig. 91) to glandular. Ventral curvature (chordee; Fig. 92) may occur on erection and is an indication for surgery. Circumcision should not be performed until reconstructive plastic surgery has been considered.

Circumcision

The prepuce is closely adherent to the glans during early childhood, and retraction is unnecessary and undesirable. Spontaneous separation occurs after some years. The only medical indications for circumcision are phimosis, paraphimosis, and recurrent balanitis.

Undescended testes

Undescended testes are common in young infants; exploration and orchidopexy are indicated if the testes fail to descend by 1 year of age. Retractile testes due to an active cremasteric reflex are extremely common and entirely normal.

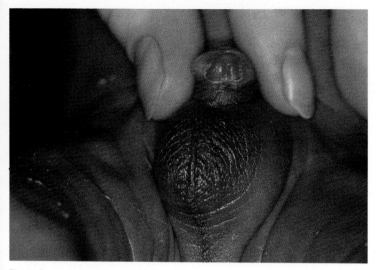

Fig. 91 Severe perineal hypospadias.

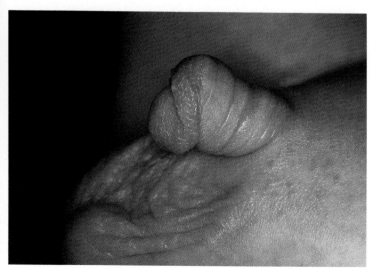

Fig. 92 Ventral curvature of penis (chordee).

Nephrotic syndrome

Incidence

1 in 20,000 children. Boys are more commonly affected. The peak age incidence is 1–5 years.

Etiology

Cause unknown; immunologic basis likely.

Clinical features

Periorbital (Fig. 93) and generalized oedema, abdominal pain and ascites. Gross proteinuria may lead to hypovolemia and acute circulatory collapse. Prone to pneumococcal peritonitis.

Management

Bed rest and high-protein, salt-restricted diet until diuresis occurs, usually within 10–14 days of starting oral corticosteroids. Hypovolemia responds to infusion of plasma or salt-free albumin.

Course and prognosis

Majority have minimal change lesion and recover completely within 2 years. Relapses are common but normally respond to steroids. Cyclophosphamide therapy is occasionally necessary.

Inguinal hernias and hydroceles

Both are due to persistent patency of the processus vaginalis. Hydroceles in the newborn usually resolve spontaneously within the first year, but in older boys, surgery will be necessary. Inguinal hernias (Fig. 94) always require surgery, and the risk of strangulation is high, particularly in young infants.

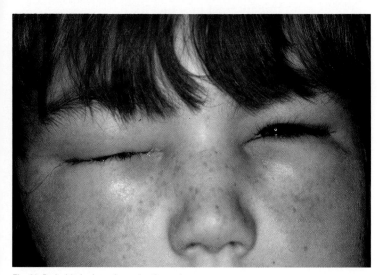

Fig. 93 Periorbital edema in nephrotic syndrome.

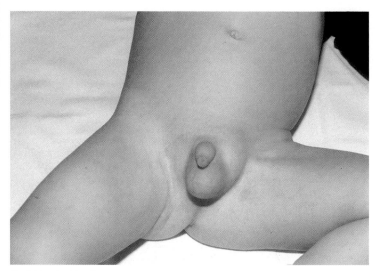

Fig. 94 Inguinal hernia.

Urinary tract infection (UTI)

Incidence
Very common infection; occurs in 1–2% of girls.

Clinical features
The young child usually has nonspecific symptoms of poor weight gain, fever, vomiting, and irritability. Older children may complain of urinary frequency, dysuria, and loin pain.

Diagnosis
High index of suspicion; must obtain adequate urine sample for urinalysis and culture. Suprapubic aspirate is often necessary in young infants because skin contamination may make bag or clean-catch specimens difficult to interpret, particularly in girls.

Management
Acute infection requires antibiotic therapy. All proven UTIs require investigation of the renal tract with ultrasound examination and sometimes intravenous urogram, radioisotope scans, or micturating cystourethrogram. At least 50% have an underlying abnormality, most commonly vesicoureteric reflux (Fig. 95). Prophylactic antibiotics may protect against renal scarring. New scars rarely develop after the age of 7 years. Surgery is occasionally necessary and usually involves ureteric reimplantation.

Renal tract anomalies

Incidence
Relatively common; most are asymptomatic and functionally insignificant.

Clinical features
Ureteric duplication is usually asymptomatic but may predispose to infection, obstruction, or reflux. Posterior urethral valves in male infants cause poor urinary stream, and obstruction may cause renal failure. Horseshoe kidneys, pelvic kidneys, and unilateral renal dysplasia are often asymptomatic unless there is infection. Severe anomalies of the renal tract such as renal agenesis or prune-belly syndrome (Fig. 96) are usually diagnosed shortly after birth.

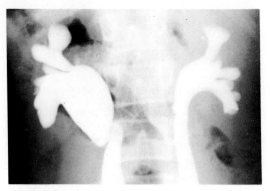

Fig. 95 Vesicoureteric reflux (bilateral grade III).

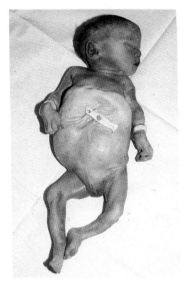

Fig. 96 Prune-belly syndrome.

Congenital heart disease

Incidence

Common; at least 1 in 300 live births.

Etiology

Usually unknown; sometimes associated with chromosomal abnormality or rubella embryopathy.

Clinical features

Asymptomatic cardiac murmurs are often heard during routine examination. Cyanosis (Fig. 97) or heart failure usually indicate a serious structural defect. Clubbing of the fingers and toes (Fig. 98) may develop in conditions such as Fallot's tetralogy when there is long-standing cyanosis.

Investigation

CXR and electrocardiograph are often helpful, but rarely diagnostic. Ultrasound examination and cardiac catheterization give more precise detail of cardiac structure. When coarctation of the aorta is suspected because of inequality or delay of femoral pulses, blood pressure must be measured and a difference between the upper and lower limbs is significant.

Management

Depends on underlying problem. The most common abnormality is a ventricular septal defect (VSD). Most VSDs close spontaneously or become functionally insignificant in later childhood. Surgery is usually required for more serious defects.

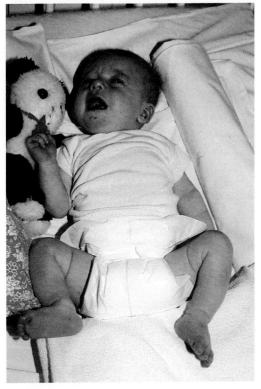

Fig. 97 Cyanotic congenital heart disease.

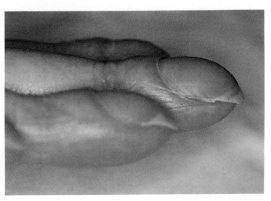

Fig. 98 Finger clubbing in cyanotic heart disease.

Bronchiolitis

Commonly occurs in infants in winter epidemics; usually due to respiratory syncytial virus.

Clinical features

Coryzal symptoms, then gradual onset of cough, wheeze, tachypnea, and feeding difficulty. The child may develop overinflation of the lungs, producing a barrel-shaped chest, cyanosis, subcostal recession (Fig. 99), and occasionally heart failure.

Management

Supportive care with added oxygen when necessary. Tube feeding or intravenous fluids are often required. Antibiotics are not usually indicated but may be given if secondary infection is suspected or in a very ill child. Treatment of cardiac failure or mechanical ventilation is occasionally necessary. A nebulized antiviral agent, ribavirin, may be indicated in high-risk babies, such as those with congenital heart disease.

Asthma

Incidence

A very common respiratory illness in childhood; one in seven children affected.

Etiology

Allergens, particularly house dust mite, are always important in children. There is often a family history of asthma, allergies, or eczema.

Clinical features

Mild asthmatics may have only chronic cough, particularly nocturnal or exercise-induced. More severe symptoms include wheezing and respiratory distress. Children with chronic undertreated asthma may develop chest deformity (Fig. 100) and growth failure.

Management

Severity of attack best assessed by monitoring peak flow. Acute bronchospasm usually responds to inhaled beta-sympathomimetics or xanthines. Prophylaxis with inhaled sodium cromoglycate or corticosteroids is helpful in chronic asthma.

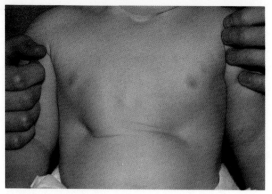

Fig. 99 Chest recession in bronchiolitis.

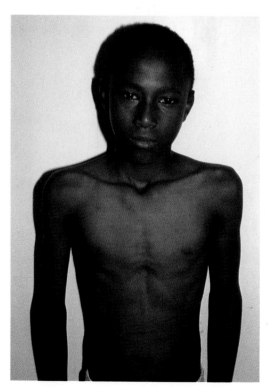

Fig. 100 Chest deformity in a chronic asthmatic child.

Acute laryngotracheobronchitis (croup)

Incidence

Common in children younger than 4 years of age. It is usually a viral illness.

Clinical features

Coryzal symptoms for several days, then development of a characteristic barking cough and inspiratory stridor (croup). Symptoms often worse at night or when child is anxious or crying. When cyanosis or subcostal recession is present, the child should be observed in hospital.

Management

There is no evidence that humidification, steroids, or antibiotics are of any value, but they are sometimes used. Oxygen should be provided when there are signs of hypoxia. Occasionally, tracheal intubation may be required if there is severe airways obstruction or exhaustion.

Acute epiglottitis

Incidence

Uncommon but potentially fatal. Occurs in children aged 4–10 years.

Etiology

Hemophilus influenzae type B infection of epiglottis.

Clinical features

Sudden onset of severe stridor and upper airways obstruction. Children rapidly become toxic and develop life-threatening obstruction within a few hours.

Management

Examination of the epiglottis should only be attempted when there is immediate expert provision for maintaining an adequate airway. Tracheal intubation (Fig. 101) is often necessary but frequently difficult. Tracheostomy (Fig. 102) is occasionally unavoidable.

Intravenous ampicillin and cefotaxime usually control the edema and inflammation of the epiglottis within a few days.

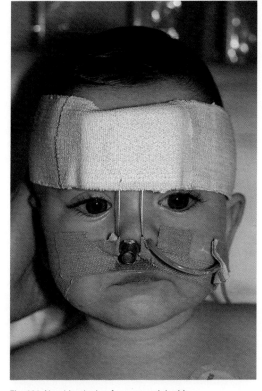

Fig. 101 Nasal intubation for acute epiglottitis.

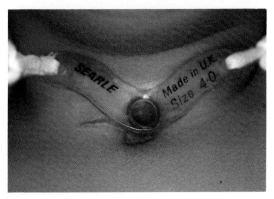

Fig. 102 Tracheostomy.

Pneumonia

Etiology

In infancy, bronchopneumonia is usually caused by *Hemophilus influenzae* or rarely by *Staphylococcus aureus*. Pneumococcal infection causes lobar pneumonia in older children. *Mycoplasma pneumoniae* is also a cause.

Clinical features

Fever, tachypnea, meningism, and feeding difficulties are common. Localizing signs are often absent in young infants, so CXR is usually necessary in any ill child (Fig. 103). Recurrent chest infections or localized airtrapping is sometimes due to inhalation of a foreign body.

Management

Broad-spectrum antibiotics until specific organism and sensitivities identified. Erythromycin is indicated when mycoplasma pneumonia is suspected.

Cystic fibrosis

Incidence

The most common cause of suppurative chronic lung disease and pancreatic insufficiency in children in the United States, the United Kingdom, and Australia. There is autosomal recessive inheritance, and the carrier rate in the general population is 1 in 20. Cystic fibrosis affects 1 in 1,600 live births.

Etiology

Abnormality of exocrine and mucus-secreting glands; the etiology is unknown. Carriers are asymptomatic and undetectable by current methods.

Clinical features

Affected neonates may have meconium ileus and gut obstruction. Usually have recurrent chest infections (Fig. 104), failure to thrive, and malabsorption within the first few years of life. Diagnosis confirmed by sweat test.

Management

Pancreatic extract supplements control the pancreatic insufficiency and malabsorption. Prompt and aggressive treatment of chest infections with antibiotics and postural drainage. Prophylactic antibiotics may be helpful. Long-term survival into adult life depends on severity of chest involvement. Chronic chest deformity and infections caused by antibiotic-resistant organisms frequently develop. Antenatal diagnosis is now possible in affected families using DNA analysis after chorionic villous sampling.

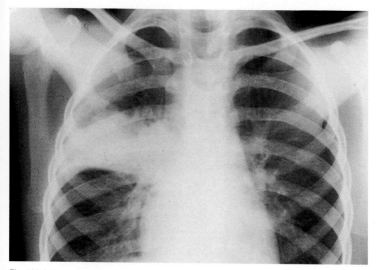

Fig. 103 Lobar pneumonia.

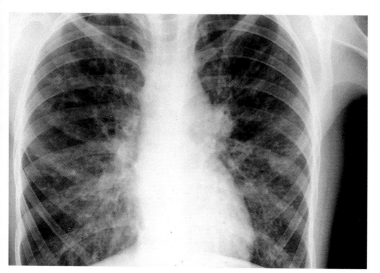

Fig. 104 Cystic fibrosis.

Meningomyelocele (spina bifida)

Management and complications

After neonatal surgery, a variety of specialist help will be required. Surgical closure of the spinal defect (Fig. 105) is usually not difficult, but long-term complications are common. Urinary incontinence and UTIs are common and distressing. Congenital dislocation of the hips and talipes equinovarus are frequent orthopedic complications. Hydrocephalus often requires insertion of a shunt.

Prognosis

Despite the long-term complications, with sympathetic and careful early assessment, many children lead rewarding and meaningful lives.

Hydrocephalus

Etiology

Congenital aqueduct stenosis; or secondary to meningitis or hemorrhage.

Clinical features

Rapid growth of cerebral ventricles and head circumference. Setting-sun eyes (Fig. 106), crack-pot percussion sign, and positive transillumination are late signs of hydrocephalus.

Management

Once the diagnosis is confirmed by serial measurements, ultrasound, or computed tomography scan, shunt surgery is usually necessary (Fig. 107).

Prognosis

With early diagnosis, the prognosis is good for uncomplicated hydrocephalus, but this depends on the underlying cause.

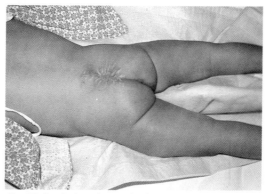

Fig. 105 Repaired meningomyelocele.

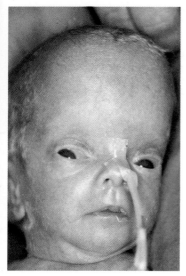

Fig. 106 Setting-sun eye sign.

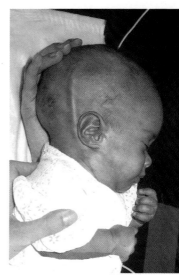

Fig. 107 Ventriculoperitoneal shunt.

Cerebral palsy

Incidence

2 per 1,000 live births.

Etiology

The precise cause is often obscure; some cases are due to anoxic brain damage in fetal or early neonatal life. It is more common in small, preterm babies.

Clinical features

Permanent but nonprogressive disorder of movement and posture. Clinical features often change because the child is continuing to grow and develop. Infants often show poor sucking, feeding difficulties, hypotonia, hypertonia, or irritability. Cerebral palsy is often not diagnosed for several months, when delayed or abnormal motor development become more obvious. About 70% of children with cerebral palsy have spastic manifestations with scissoring of legs (Fig. 108), opisthotonos, hypertonia, clonus, and brisk tendon reflexes. One or several limbs may be involved, giving rise to hemiplegia, diplegia, or quadriplegia. Ataxic cerebral palsy with hypotonia and weakness occurs in approximately 10%. Choreoathetosis characterized by irregular involuntary movements accounts for another 10% and is sometimes associated with hyperbilirubinemia (kernicterus).

Complications

Mental retardation, epilepsy, and sensory handicap are present in at least 60% of children with cerebral palsy.

Management

A multidisciplinary approach to assessment and long-term management is essential. Physiotherapy may encourage normal motor development and prevent contractures. The "wind-swept" deformity (Fig. 109) seen after prolonged immobilization should be avoidable.

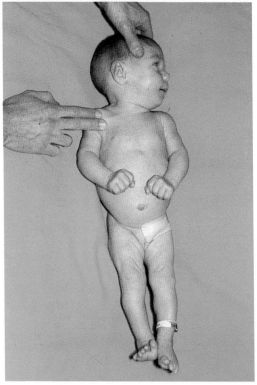

Fig. 108 Scissoring of legs.

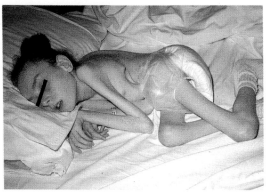

Fig. 109 "Wind-swept" deformity.

Duchenne muscular dystrophy

Incidence
The most common muscular dystrophy; occurs in 1 in 4,000 male infants.

Inheritance
Sex-linked recessive, but mutations are frequent. Female carriers are often asymptomatic but can often be identified.

Clinical features
Usually presents within the first 5 years because of difficulty in climbing stairs and frequent falls. The calf muscles are prominent (Fig. 110) but weak. When attempting to rise to standing from sitting or lying position, the boy "climbs up" his legs using his hands for support (Gower's sign).

Diagnosis
Elevated CPK; abnormal electromyograph and muscle biopsy.

Course and prognosis
Progressive weakness resulting in most boys being confined to a wheelchair by teenage years. Death, usually from respiratory infections, occurs in early adult life.

Antenatal diagnosis
An affected male fetus can be identified using DNA analysis. Carrier females can be identified in some cases by a mildly elevated CPK.

Werdnig–Hoffmann disease (spinal muscular atrophy)

Incidence
Occurs in 1 in 20,000 live births.

Inheritance
Autosomal recessive inheritance.

Clinical features
Infants are often weak and floppy from birth (Fig. 111). Rapidly progressive with death from respiratory failure within 12–18 months.

Antenatal diagnosis
Now available for some affected families.

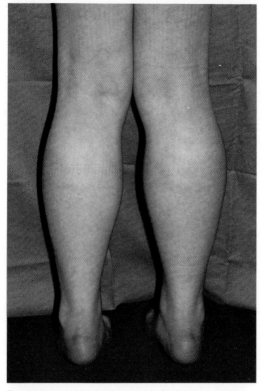

Fig. 110 Hypertrophied calf muscles in Duchenne muscular dystrophy.

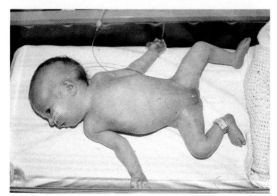

Fig. 111 Frog-like posture of infant with Werdnig–Hoffmann disease.

The floppy baby

Etiology

Describes clinical condition of hypotonic infant in first year of life. There are many possible underlying causes. Paralytic causes include neuromuscular disorders and cerebral palsy. Non-paralytic causes are hypothyroidism, malnutrition, and Down syndrome. A few floppy infants have delayed but eventually normal motor development (benign congenital hypotonia). Benign hypotonia is often familial.

Clinical features

A useful method of assessment is to hold the young infant in ventral suspension and pull the infant from supine to sitting posture (Fig. 112).

Arthrogryposis multiplex congenita

Clinical features

Clinical syndrome in which there are flexion contractures of muscles and joints, gross muscle wasting, and sometimes dislocation of joints (Fig. 113).

Etiology

Usually unknown, may have primary muscle hypoplasia. Sometimes secondary to constricted intrauterine position because of oligohydramnios or uterine abnormality.

Management

Long-term physiotherapy may improve contractures. Surgery often helpful later. Long-term prognosis depends on severity of muscular hypoplasia.

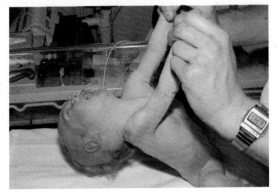

Fig. 112 Marked head lag of floppy newborn infant.

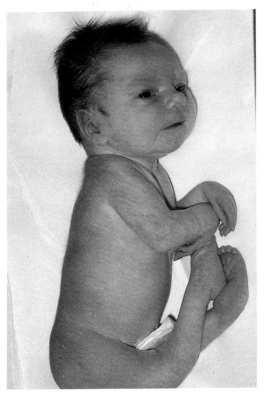

Fig. 113 Arthrogryposis multiplex congenita.

Poliomyelitis

Uncommon in countries with successful immunization policy.

Initially a mild viral illness with fever, sore throat, headache, and vomiting, lasting several days. About 1 week later, in approximately 30% of cases, there are more severe symptoms of headache, neck stiffness, leg and back pains, and progressive asymmetrical weakness with muscular paralysis due to anterior horn cell damage.

In severe cases, death may occur from respiratory failure and bulbar paralysis in the acute illness. In the majority, there is gradual improvement over 12–18 months. Many children have residual muscle wasting and paralysis (Fig. 114).

Neurofibromatosis

Von Recklinghausen's disease.

1 in 3,000 live births.

Autosomal dominant; but at least 50% due to new mutation.

Most have areas of skin hypo- or hyperpigmentation (café-au-lait spots) (Fig. 115). Pigmented spots in the axillae are characteristic. Subcutaneous fibromata, neurofibromata of peripheral nerves and viscera are common. Many have skeletal abnormalities and pseudoarthroses.

Pheochromocytoma and glioma are common. At least 50% develop some neurologic impairment.

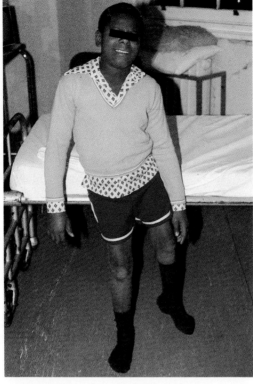

Fig. 114 Old poliomyelitis with shortening of leg.

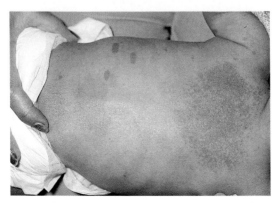

Fig. 115 Café-au-lait spots, pigmented lesions, and shagreen patch in neurofibromatosis.

Myasthenia gravis

Incidence	Uncommon in early childhood. Peak incidence in adolescent girls.
Etiology	Autoimmune disorder; anticholinesterase antibodies can be demonstrated in majority.
Clinical features	Gradual onset of muscle weakness, with early fatigue. Loss of facial expression, arm weakness, chewing difficulty, and ptosis (Fig. 116) are common. Transient form of myasthenia gravis occurs in infants of mothers with the disease due to transplacental passage of antibodies.
Diagnosis	Clinically confirmed by showing prompt improvement with intravenous edrophonium (Tensilon) (Fig. 117).
Management	Long-acting anticholinesterase drugs such as pyridostigmine. Thymectomy often helpful.

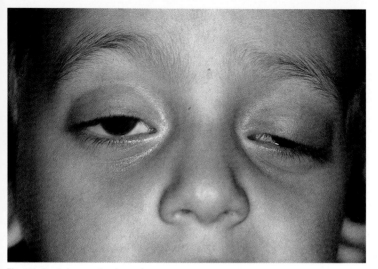

Fig. 116 Ptosis in myasthenia gravis.

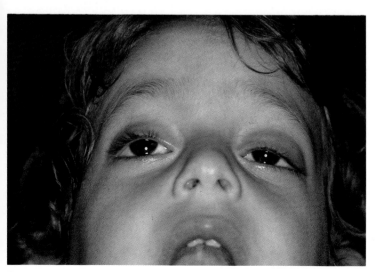

Fig. 117 Improvement after intravenous edrophonium.

Arthritis

Pyogenic arthritis

Usually a single, hot, swollen, tender joint with painful restriction of movement. *Staphylococcus aureus* is the most common infective organism. Surgical drainage is often necessary for diagnosis and treatment.

Rheumatic fever

There has been a dramatic reduction in the incidence of this disease in developed countries. Classically, there is an acute migratory polyarthritis associated with fever, rash, and sometimes subcutaneous nodules. Carditis is the most serious long-term complication, resulting in permanent valvular damage.

Henoch–Schönlein purpura

A common allergic vasculitis that causes an easily recognizable clinical picture. There is a characteristic purpuric rash (see Figs. 67–69), flitting arthritis or arthralgia, abdominal pain, and hematuria. The majority resolve rapidly and require only rest and analgesia.

Juvenile rheumatoid arthritis (JRA)

Peak incidence of systemic disease is 1–5 years of age. Recurrent painful swelling and stiffness of both small (Fig. 118) and large joints (Figs. 119 and 120) is common in older children. Weight loss and mild anemia are associated findings. Joint inflammation can be reduced by appropriate choice of anti-inflammatory drugs. Exercise, physiotherapy, hydrotherapy, and night splints help to limit deformity. Acute inflammatory episodes often remit spontaneously but sometimes only after many years.

Common clinical types

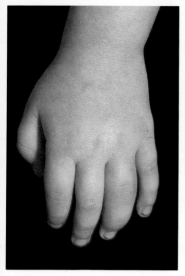

Fig. 118 Swelling of small joints of the hand in JRA. (By courtesy of Dr. B. Ansell.)

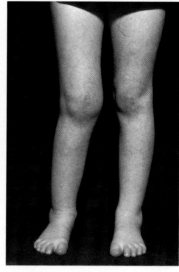

Fig. 119 Monoarthritis of knee. (By courtesy of Dr. B. Ansell.)

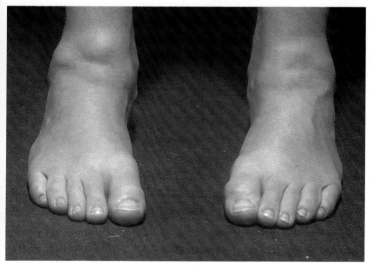

Fig. 120 Gross swelling of ankles. (By courtesy of Dr. B. Ansell.)

Leukemia

Incidence

The most common childhood malignancy; 85% have acute lymphoblastic leukemia (ALL).

Clinical features

Pallor, lethargy, recurrent infections, fever, and spontaneous bruising are common. Hepatosplenomegaly, lymphadenopathy, and bone tenderness sometimes occur.

Diagnosis

Neonatal leukemia, although rare, may present with characteristic subcutaneous deposits (Fig. 121). Anemia, thrombocytopenia, and blast cells in peripheral blood. Excessive blast cells in bone marrow confirm the diagnosis.

Management

Full discussion of treatment and prognosis with the family is very important. Transfusions of blood, platelets, or granulocytes are often necessary. Maintenance chemotherapy with several cytotoxic drugs will continue for several years. Bone marrow transplantation is becoming an important method of treatment.

Prognosis

At least 70% 5-year survival now occurs in ALL.

Histiocytosis

Pathology

Abnormal proliferation of histiocytes; variable disease spectrum that sometimes runs malignant course.

Clinical features

Clearly defined lytic bone lesions, often involving the skull, are usually benign (eosinophilic granuloma). Systemic disease with fever, hepatosplenomegaly, lymphadenopathy, seborrheic rash, or skin deposits (Figs. 122 and 123) is more serious.

Management

Systemic disease may respond to cytotoxic chemotherapy similar to treatment for acute leukemia.

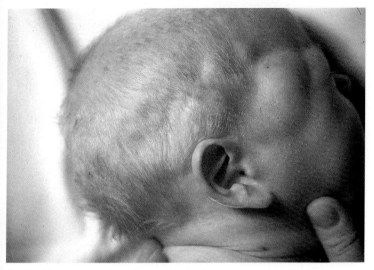

Fig. 121 Subcutaneous lesions of neonatal leukemia.

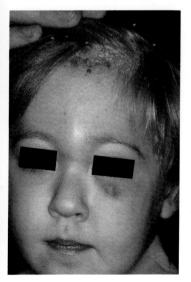

Fig. 122 Histiocytosis—skin and scalp lesions.

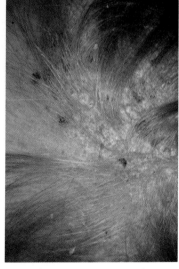

Fig. 123 Seborrheic scalp lesions of histiocytosis.

Wilms tumor (nephroblastoma)

Clinical features

Most are found as an asymptomatic abdominal mass (Fig. 124). Hematuria and abdominal pain are sometimes present.

Diagnosis

Ultrasound examination of kidney or intravenous urogram show distortion of the pelvicalyceal system.

Management and prognosis

Chemotherapy reduces the size of the tumor mass before surgery is performed. Postoperative radiotherapy is sometimes given. Overall 5-year survival is at least 80%. Metastases are often present at the time of diagnosis but frequently respond to chemotherapy or irradiation.

Neuroblastoma

Clinical features

Usually present as abdominal mass indistinguishable from Wilms tumor on clinical examination.

Diagnosis

Abdominal radiograph may show tumor calcification. Adrenal tumors displace the kidney but do not usually distort the pelvicalyceal system on intravenous urogram or ultrasound examination. Elevated urinary catecholamine levels (VMA and HVA) confirm the diagnosis in 90% of cases and are also a sensitive indicator of recurrence. Bony metastases (Fig. 125) sometimes occur.

Management and prognosis

Surgical excision followed by radiotherapy. 5-year survival is 60%; occasional spontaneous recovery reported.

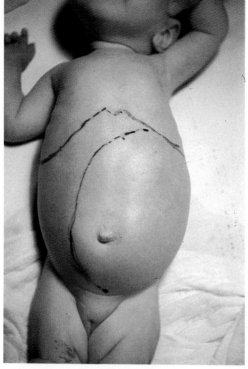

Fig. 124 Wilms tumor presenting as abdominal distension.

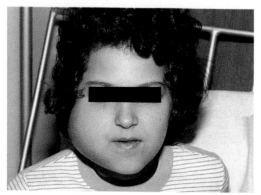

Fig. 125 Secondary neuroblastoma of mandible.

Cerebral tumor

Incidence

Second most common childhood malignancy. Most are located in the posterior fossa.

Clinical features

Headache, vomiting, ataxia, or visual disturbance are common presenting symptoms. Behavioral disturbance, mood change, or convulsions sometimes occur. Cranial nerve palsies (Fig. 126) are often found in brainstem tumors.

Management and prognosis

Surgical resection when possible, but this is often difficult or incomplete. Medulloblastomas are often radiosensitive, and 5-year survival is now at least 60%. Long-term complications of the tumor or treatment, particularly growth and endocrine disturbance, are almost invariable in survivors.

Other malignancy

Solid tumors are uncommon in childhood, but retinoblastoma, rhabdomyosarcoma, osteosarcoma, Hodgkin's disease, and lymphoma (Fig. 127) may occur. Bilateral retinoblastoma has a strong familial incidence and a good prognosis for survival with early treatment.

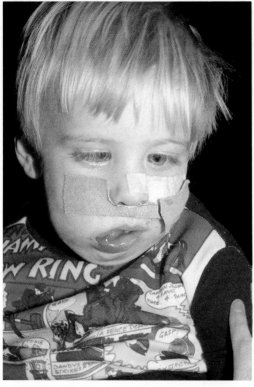

Fig. 126 VI and VII nerve palsies due to brainstem glioma.

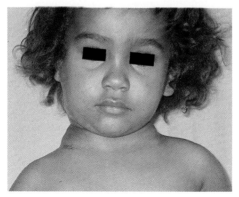

Fig. 127 Hodgkin's lymphoma.

Thalassemia

Inheritance

Autosomal recessive; each pregnancy from parents with thalassemia minor (heterozygous) carries a one in four risk of producing homozygous major disease in the infant.

Etiology

Failure of synthesis of α- or β-globin chains.

Clinical features

α-thalassemia is more common in Asians. Homozygous α-thalassemia results in hydrops fetalis with intrauterine or early neonatal death. β-Thalassemia occurs mainly in Mediterranean populations. When fetal hemoglobin (HbF) levels decline after the first few months, the child develops severe anemia, hepatosplenomegaly due to extramedullary hemopoiesis, and sometimes cardiac failure. Compensatory bone marrow hyperplasia produces characteristic expansion of the skull and facial bones in older children (Fig. 128). Skull radiographs show the characteristic hair-on-end appearance.

Management

Regular blood transfusions are necessary thoughout life.

Complications

Frequent transfusions cause chronic iron overload. Continuous subcutaneous infusions of an iron chelating agent (desferrioxamine) may improve survival. Death, usually secondary to cardiomyopathy, occurs in early adult life. Growth and puberty failure, diabetes mellitus, skin pigmentation (Fig. 129), and liver damage are other manifestations of chronic iron overload.

Antenatal diagnosis

Affected fetuses may be detected by analysis of globin chain synthesis of fetal blood, or more recently, DNA analysis of chorionic villous samples.

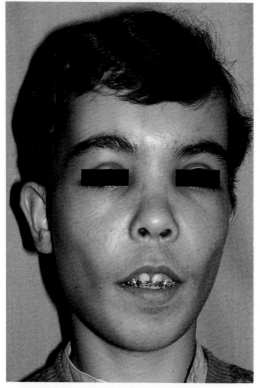

Fig. 128 Bone hyperplasia in β-thalassemia intermedia.

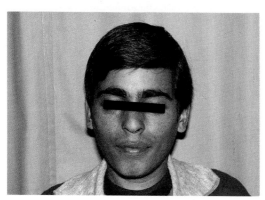

Fig. 129 Skin pigmentation in thalassemia.

Sickle cell disease

Etiology

Common. Hemoglobinopathy with sickle cell trait is found in 15% of blacks. Inheritance is autosomal recessive.

Clinical features

Chronic anemia, recurrent bone pains with tenderness and swelling, fever, and jaundice (Fig. 130). Chronic leg ulcers, hematuria, chest and abdominal pain are common.

Management

Symptomatic treatment of painful crises. Prompt antibiotic treatment of infection. Prophylactic penicillin and pneumococcal vaccines are needed to prevent serious pneumococcal infections.

Idiopathic thrombocytopenic purpura (ITP)

Etiology

Often occurs after viral infections, especially rubella. Platelet antibodies are usually detectable.

Clinical features

Spontaneous petechiae and superficial bruising (Fig. 131). Other, more serious, causes of thrombocytopenia must be excluded.

Prognosis

Majority recover spontaneously within a few months; occasionally chronic, requiring splenectomy.

Management

Platelet transfusions may be needed when the count falls to less than 10×10^3/L. Steroids and intravenous gamma globulins may also be helpful.

Bleeding disorders

Etiology

Hemophilia A (factor VIII deficiency) is the most common.

Clinical features

Spontaneous bruising or excessive bleeding after minimal trauma producing hemarthrosis (Fig. 132), deep hematomas, or mucosal hemorrhage.

Management

All trauma and surgical procedures must be treated with intravenous factor concentrates. Chronic joint damage can be reduced with early treatment of trauma and bleeding.

Antenatal diagnosis

Factor assay of fetal blood sample.

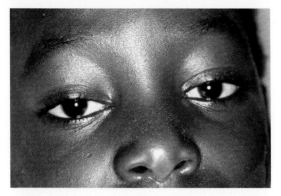

Fig. 130 Jaundiced sclera in sickle cell anemia.

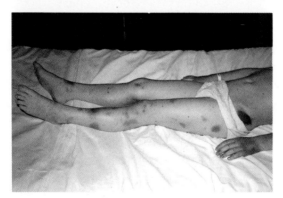

Fig. 131 Bruising in ITP.

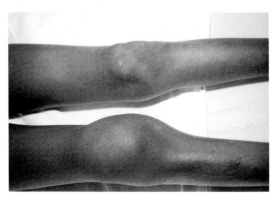

Fig. 132 Hemarthrosis in hemophilia. (By courtesy of Dr. A. Kilby.)

Bat ears

Inheritance

Often autosomal dominant.

Clinical features

Large protruding ears, usually bilateral (Fig. 133).

Pathology

Defect in the normal folding process of the anti-helix.

Significance and treatment

Corrective surgery when protrusion of ears is cosmetically unacceptable.

Torticollis

Etiology

Usually acute onset of unknown etiology. Chronic painless torticollis may be secondary to sternomastoid fibrosis, intrauterine posture, cervical hemivertebrae, or ocular imbalance.

Clinical features

In acute painful torticollis or the common wryneck (Fig. 134), there is a sudden onset of limitation of neck rotation with an intensely painful sternomastoid muscle. The head is sometimes tilted toward the affected side.

Management

Spontaneous recovery occurs within days in acute torticollis or months in postural torticollis. Gentle physiotherapy may be helpful.

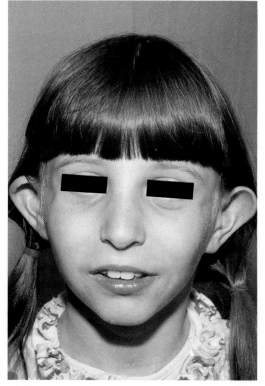

Fig. 133 Bat ears.

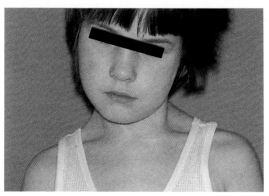

Fig. 134 Acute torticollis.

Cleft lip and palate

Management

Cleft lip (Fig. 135) is repaired as early as possible, and the palate within the first year of life. Further plastic surgery to elevate the alae nasi to improve the cosmetic appearance is sometimes necessary in later childhood (Fig. 136). Additional specialist help may be required to deal with orthodontic problems, speech difficulties, and eustachian tube obstruction.

Choanal atresia

Incidence

Rare anomaly in which there is absence or narrowing of the posterior nares. May occur as part of the CHARGE association (colobomas, heart defect, atresia choanae, mental and growth retardation, genital hypoplasia, ear anomalies).

Clinical features

Bilateral choanal atresia causes cyanosis and respiratory obstruction in the newborn. In unilateral choanal atresia, the condition causes unilateral rhinorrhea, and diagnosis is often not made until later in childhood.

Management

Urgent provision of an oral airway is needed in bilateral choanal atresia. The membranous posterior nares are then surgically excised and a small tube left in situ until the new orifice has epithelialized (Fig. 137).

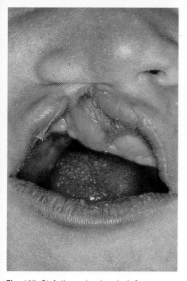

Fig. 135 Cleft lip and palate in infancy.

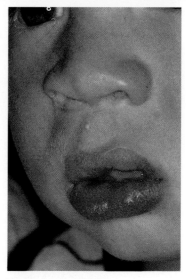

Fig. 136 Repaired cleft lip.

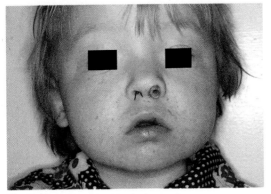

Fig. 137 Choanal atresia with tube in nostril.

Developmental limb anomalies (1)

Common, particularly anomalies of the hand and arms.

Usually unknown. Absent radius or limb reduction defects may occur after a major vascular catastrophe in fetal life. Phocomelia is known to occur with maternal ingestion of drugs such as thalidomide in early pregnancy.

Extra digits (polydactyly) of the hands and feet (Fig. 138) are extremely common and are often of autosomal dominant inheritance. Extra digits on the hand usually require surgical excision in early life. Polydactyly of the toes may require excision when the provision of comfortable footwear is difficult when the child is older.

Syndactyly (Fig. 139) particularly of the second and third toes is extremely common and is never of any functional significance.

Absent radius and thumb (Fig. 140) is sometimes found in association with thrombocytopenia or anemia. ➡

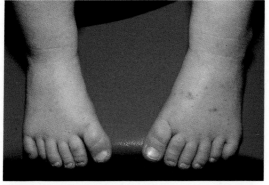

Fig. 138 Polydactyly of toes.

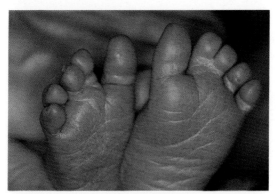

Fig. 139 Syndactyly of second and third toes.

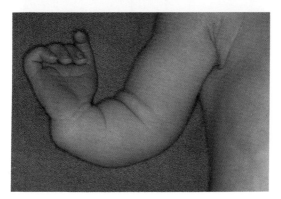

Fig. 140 Absent radius and thumb.

Developmental limb anomalies (2)

Clinical features (cont.)

Missing digits (Fig. 141) sometimes occur.

Complete absence of the hand (Fig. 142) is the most common limb reduction deformity. Sometimes almost the whole limb is missing (Fig. 143). The etiology is usually obscure. Prosthetic substitutes should be provided before the age of acquisition of skills requiring hand coordination.

Claw hand (Fig. 144) and foot are uncommon anomalies of major functional significance. Surgery is usually considered but is not always necessary.

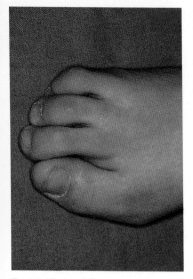

Fig. 141 Missing digit.

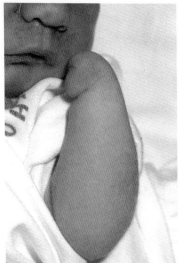

Fig. 142 Limb reduction deformity with absent hand.

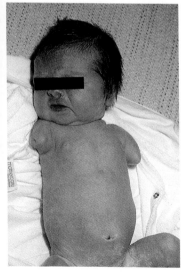

Fig. 143 Missing limbs in a newborn.

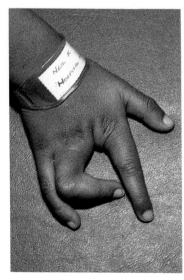

Fig. 144 Claw hand.

Postural deformities of the leg and foot

Common clinical types

Bow legs
In the first 2 years of life, the tibia of the normal child has an outward curve and internal rotation. This bow-legged appearance (Fig. 145) is often more apparent when walking begins. Spontaneous improvement occurs.

Knock-knees
After 2 years of age, there may be unequal growth of the femoral condyles, which gives rise to the knock-knee posture (genu valgum) (Fig. 146). Girls are more commonly affected.

Gradual improvement occurs, and by 6–7 years of age the legs are usually straight.

In-toeing
The most common cause is metatarsus varus. The feet tend to curve medially because of adduction of the forefoot (Fig. 147). The natural tendency is for improvement with growth, although surgery is occasionally necessary. Excessive internal rotation of the femora is common in girls and this also causes in-toeing. Treatment is unnecessary because spontaneous resolution occurs.

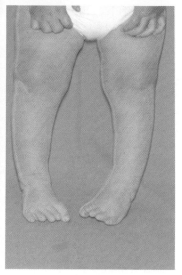

Fig. 145 Normal bow legs in infancy.

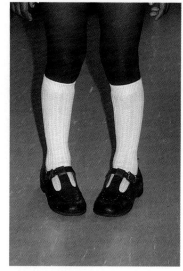

Fig. 146 Knock-knee.

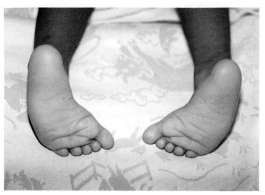

Fig. 147 Metatarsus varus.

Scoliosis

Etiology

Usually idiopathic; occurs mainly in adolescent girls.

Clinical features

Spinal curvature is best detected by asking the child to bend forward with the arms hanging freely. Usually asymptomatic but can progress to severe cosmetic deformity. Severe scoliosis may cause respiratory embarrassment or spinal cord complications. Midline lesions, such as hemangiomas (Fig. 148), hairy nevi, or lipomas, may indicate an underlying vertebral anomaly, particularly when they occur in the lumbosacral region.

Management

Bracing or surgical correction may be necessary when deformity progresses.

Hip disorders

Incidence and etiology

The most common cause of limp or hip pain is transient synovitis (irritable hip) or trauma. Avascular necrosis of the femoral head (Perthes' disease) occurs in boys aged 5–10 years. Etiology is unknown. Obese teenage boys occasionally develop slipped upper femoral epiphyses.

Clinical features

Usually sudden onset of limp and hip pain. There is restriction of abduction, extension, and internal rotation.

Diagnosis

Radiographs are diagnostic in Perthes' disease (Fig. 149) and slipped femoral epiphyses. Irritable hip is diagnosed after exclusion of infection and specific joint and bone disorders.

Management

Irritable hip recovers with a few days or weeks of bed rest. Limb traction, surgery, or internal fixation may be necessary in Perthes' disease and slipped femoral epiphyses.

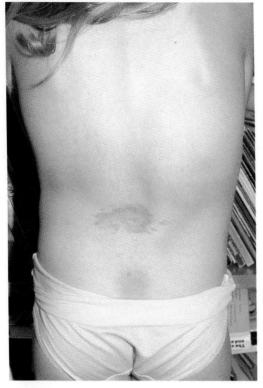

Fig. 148 Scoliosis and midline hemangioma.

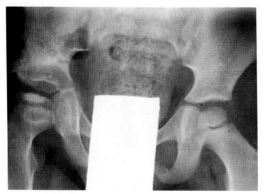

Fig. 149 Radiograph of Perthes' disease.

Cystic hygroma

Clinical features

Most become apparent in the first year of life. The hygroma is a developmental anomaly of the lymphatic channels, which gives rise to an ill-defined fluctuant cystic mass (Fig. 150), usually in the neck. Today, they are often recognized antenatally by ultrasound. They may be associated with Turner syndrome, and peripheral lymphedema may also be present.

Management

Surgical excision is necessary as the mass slowly enlarges, causing cosmetic embarrassment, and occasionally becomes infected or causes respiratory distress.

Lipoma

Incidence

Common.

Clinical features

Soft subcutaneous mass (Fig. 151), which may be located anywhere on the body. Can usually be distinguished from lymphangiomas, which transilluminate.

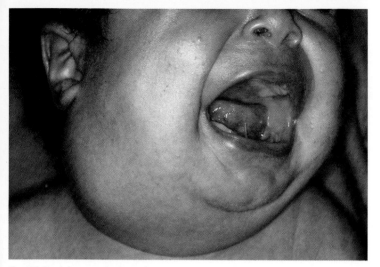

Fig. 150 Cystic hygroma in the neck.

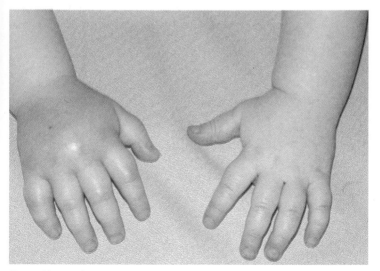

Fig. 151 Lipoma of hand.

Fractures

Clinical features

Pain, swelling, and loss of function of a limb. A history of trauma is not always obtained, particularly in the very young.

Management

Exact anatomic reposition is not always necessary in children, as efficient remodeling ensures a good end result. Fracture of the humerus in young infants (usually due to birth trauma) requires only a collar-and-cuff sling. Callus formation and healing are more rapid in young children. Even a major fracture of the femur will heal rapidly after a few weeks of immobilization in gallows traction (Fig. 152).

Complications

Arterial ischemia (Fig. 154) or nerve injury is the major complication of any fracture.

Osteogenesis imperfecta

Clinical features

The severe congenital form is usually lethal in utero or shortly after birth. In the later onset type of osteogenesis imperfecta, fractures occur spontaneously or with minimal trauma.

Complications

Severe chest and limb deformity (Fig. 153) may result if fractures are not recognized and treated appropriately. Although the frequency of fractures decreases with age, the child usually has short stature and some permanent deformity and disability in later life. Progressive deafness may also occur.

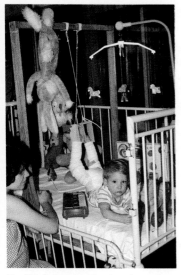

Fig. 152 Gallows traction. Legs in traction but still partly mobile!

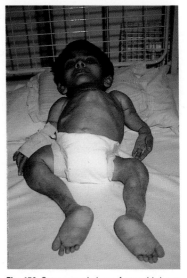

Fig. 153 Osteogenesis imperfecta with bony deformity.

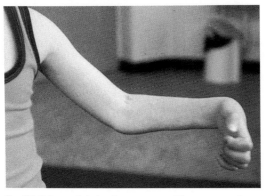

Fig. 154 Volkmann's ischemic contracture of forearm secondary to supracondylar fracture of humerus. (By courtesy of Dr. A. Kilby.)

Burns and scalds

Clinical features

The most common scald happens to the toddler who pulls boiling water onto the face, neck, shoulder, and upper arm (Fig. 155). Flame burns tend to happen to older children. When clothes catch fire, burns may involve extensive areas of the body (Fig. 156) and are often deep.

Management

Treatment depends on the extent and severity of the burn. Emergency measures consist of pain relief (particularly for superficial scalds), ensuring an adequate airway, and resuscitation with plasma volume expanders when there are signs of shock. If burns involve more than 10% of the child's surface area, intravenous therapy will be necessary. Large quantities of fluid, blood, and protein are lost from burned areas. Tetanus toxoid should always be given. Infection should be prevented by barrier nursing of exposed burns or by the closed method with topical antibiotics such as silver sulfadiazine under occlusive dressings (Fig. 157). Systemic antibiotics are given if there are specific indications.

Course and prognosis

Superficial burns quickly form a protective eschar when left exposed. This eschar gradually lifts off when new epithelium has formed (Fig. 158). Skin grafts may be necessary for deep or extensive burns or to relieve tight contractures.

Prevention

Burns should be preventable by education of the public and safeguards in design of heating appliances and children's clothing.

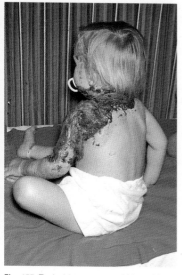

Fig. 155 Typical hot water scald in toddler.

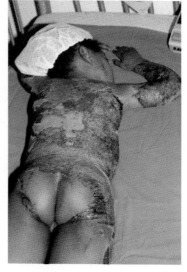

Fig. 156 Extensive flame burns.

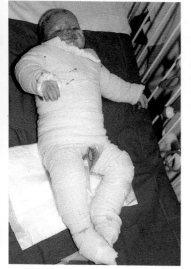

Fig. 157 Extensive burns treated by closed dressings.

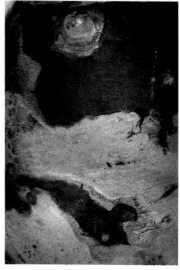

Fig. 158 New epithelium forming after a scald.

13 / Nonaccidental injury

Etiology

Nonaccidental injury or child abuse usually occurs when parents or child caregivers injure their dependent but demanding child. Child abuse may also take the more subtle form of neglect or deprivation.

Clinical features

There is often a history of supposed accident. Suspicion should be aroused when history and injury are conflicting, inconsistent, or repeated. Unexplained fractures or bruises, particularly multiple or of varying age, are often found. Rough handling or direct hitting may cause fractures of ribs or long bones. Gripping and shaking an infant may leave finger-mark bruises. Shaken infants often have retinal hemorrhages. Cigarette burns (Fig. 159) leave discrete punched-out lesions. Whip marks (Fig. 160) are more common in older children. Dip burns to the buttocks and feet (Fig. 161) occur when an infant is lowered into scalding water. Human bite marks (Fig. 162) are sometimes clearly seen.

Management

If nonaccidental injury is suspected, society has a responsibility to protect the child. In addition to medical treatment of the injuries, this will involve assessment of the family situation and possible contributing factors and exclusion of alternative diagnoses. With careful supervision and sympathetic support, many children can continue to be cared for by their parents. Occasionally, the child may be safer in the care of others.

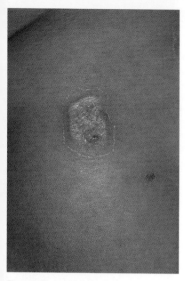

Fig. 159 Cigarette burn.

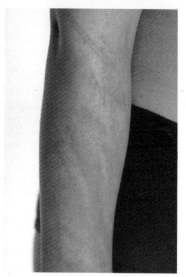

Fig. 160 Whip marks.

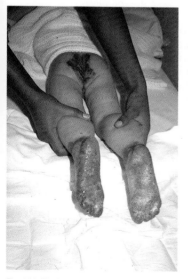

Fig. 161 Dip burns.

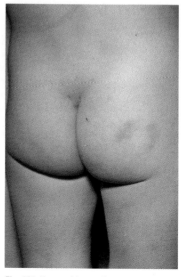

Fig. 162 Human bite marks.

It has been recognized with increasing frequency recently. Only a few are associated with a sudden or violent attack. In most cases, the children have been abused by somebody in the family or known to the child; therefore acute injury is uncommon.

Presentation

It is important that a child who gives a suspicious history of abuse is believed. Children may present with many minor symptoms including vaginal discharge, vaginal bleeding, UTI, abdominal pain, or perineal soreness and irritation. A change in behavior may be extremely significant.

Physical signs

The majority show no abnormal physical signs, but there are important pointers to the diagnosis even though they occur in only 10–30% of cases. Visible bruising in the perineal region and a torn hymen, although uncommon, may be diagnostic of violent abuse. Most vaginal discharge is not due to sexually transmitted infection, but occasionally gonorrhea may be diagnosed on culture (Fig. 163). Other infections, such as genital warts, can be caught venerally (Fig. 164), but proving that this was due to child sexual abuse is difficult because there may be other methods of transmission of the human papillomavirus.

Whenever there is vulval bleeding or soreness, a careful inspection should be made to see if there are signs such as gaping vagina or anus. The limits of normality are difficult to define; always ask an experienced clinician to make an assessment if in doubt. Other medical conditions, lichen sclerosus et atrophicus (Fig. 165) or rare conditions such as vulval psoriasis (Fig. 166), may be mistaken for child sexual abuse.

Management

Management of suspected child sexual abuse requires great skill. A senior and experienced clinician must be involved and appropriate consultations made with the police and social services. Long-term family therapy or individual counseling is often needed to support children and families. Legal steps are often required to protect the child.

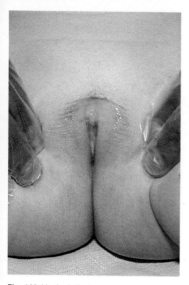

Fig. 163 Vaginal discharge.

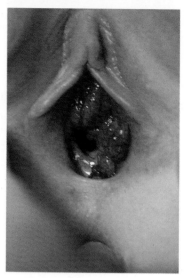

Fig. 164 Genital warts.

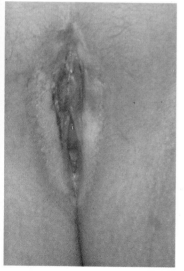

Fig. 165 Lichen sclerosus et atrophicus.

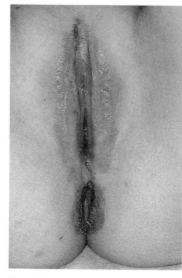

Fig. 166 Vulval psoriasis.

Congenital anomalies

Congenital ptosis

Often familial and usually unilateral (Fig. 167). In most cases, binocular vision is unaffected. Shortening of the levator palpebrae superioris may improve the cosmetic appearance or improve vision if ptosis is severe and the eyelid covers the pupil.

Microphthalmos

Developmental anomaly often associated with congenital rubella. If the palpebral fissure is short (Fig. 168), surgery may improve the cosmetic appearance.

Coloboma

Developmental anomaly of the iris (Fig. 169); often familial. Vision is usually unaffected. It is occasionally associated with a retinal anomaly.

External angular dermoid

Commonly found around the orbit, usually above and lateral to the palpebral fissure (see Fig. 71, p. 52). Surgery is usually necessary to improve appearance, because the cysts gradually increase in size.

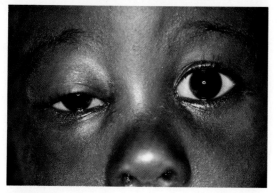

Fig. 167 Congenital ptosis.

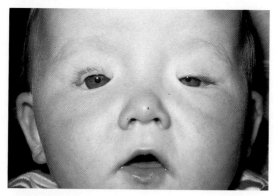

Fig. 168 Microphthalmos and ptosis.

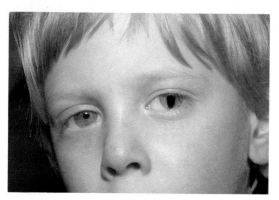

Fig. 169 Coloboma.

Strabismus (squint)

Incidence

Common in early childhood. All fixed squints and any squint that persists after 5–6 months of age require careful evaluation.

Etiology

Usually due to failure of development of binocular coordination of unknown etiology.

Clinical features

The diagnosis is usually obvious on clinical examination (Fig. 170). Symmetrical corneal reflection or occlusion testing may assist diagnosis in less obvious cases. Epicanthic folds may give rise to a false appearance of squint.

Management and prognosis

Suppression of vision (amblyopia) in the deviated eye may be permanent if squint is not detected and treated early. Correction of refractive error and occlusion of the nonsquinting eye are mandatory. Surgery is sometimes necessary.

Infection

Conjunctivitis is common in the neonatal period. Recurrent mild conjunctivitis (Fig. 171) is usually due to nonpatency of the nasolacrimal duct, which resolves towards the end of the first year of life.

Trauma

Painful corneal abrasions are usually caused by foreign bodies in the eye. Lacerations of the eyelid (Fig. 172) and penetrating eye injuries are usually the result of direct trauma.

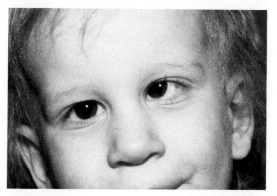

Fig. 170 Squint.

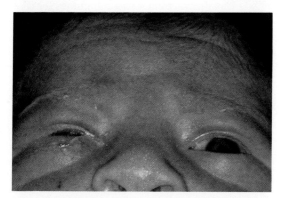

Fig. 171 Recurrent minor conjunctivitis.

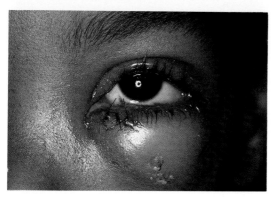

Fig. 172 Traumatic eye lesion with laceration and conjunctival hemorrhage.

Congenital glaucoma

Incidence and etiology

This congenital condition produces increased pressure inside the eye from lack of drainage at the angle of anterior chamber.

Clinical features

The eye becomes large (buphthalmos). It can be recognized in a young infant by noticing a very wide diameter of the cornea (Fig. 173). When this is greater than 11 mm, an examination by an ophthalmologist is indicated because surgery can save the child's sight. In extreme cases, the cornea becomes cloudy and may even be totally opaque.

Cataract

Etiology

Usually congenital and sometimes familial. Secondary cataracts occur in rubella embryopathy, galactosemia, and diabetes.

Clinical features

An opacity is seen in the lens (Fig. 174). Other ocular anomalies such as nystagmus or visual disturbance are often present.

Management

Depends on cause and interference with vision. Early surgery within the first month diminishes the risk of subsequent amblyopia.

Malignancy

Etiology

Retinoblastoma is the most common malignant intraocular tumor in childhood. It sometimes has autosomal dominant inheritance.

Clinical features

Opacity of the pupil, squint, or poor vision in the affected eye. Proptosis (Fig. 175) occurs with tumors involving the orbit, particularly metastatic neuroblastoma. A loss of the red reflex may be associated with retinoblastoma.

Management

Local treatment of retinoblastoma may include surgery, radiotherapy, and cryotherapy. Metastases are rare, and long-term prognosis is good.

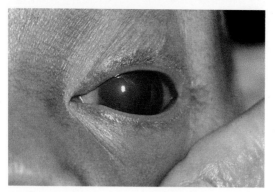

Fig. 173 Cloudy large cornea in congenital glaucoma.

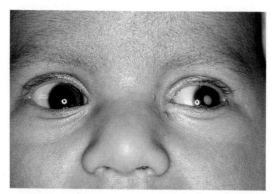

Fig. 174 Cataract.

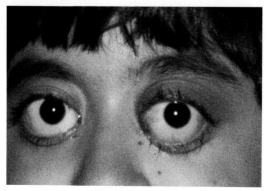

Fig. 175 Bilateral proptosis.

Down syndrome

Synonym

Trisomy 21; used to be called "mongolism".

Incidence

1 in 600 live births. The majority are due to trisomy 21, while 3% are due to translocation. There is an increased risk of trisomy 21 with increased maternal age.

Clinical features

Characteristic facial appearance (Fig. 176), hypotonia, low birth weight, and growth retardation. Prominent epicanthic folds, Brushfield's spots, and single transverse palmar creases (simian crease) are often present but also occur in 18% of normal children.

Course and prognosis

Mental retardation always occurs but varies in severity. Many of these children are now educated in normal schools. There is a high mortality in the first year due to congenital heart disease and respiratory infection. Antenatal diagnosis is possible by culture of amniotic fluid cells or chorionic villous biopsy. Women at high risk may be identified by a combination of biochemical tests on the mother's blood.

Turner syndrome

Incidence

Monosomic X syndrome with ovarian dysgenesis occurs in 1 in 5,000 live births.

Clinical features

Short stature, webbing of the neck, and failure of secondary sexual development (Fig. 177). Coarctation of the aorta occurs in girls and pulmonary stenosis is often found in boys with similar physical characteristics (Noonan syndrome).

Management

Cyclical estrogen replacement will promote secondary sexual development in adolescence, but infertility is invariable. Growth hormone is used to improve the short stature.

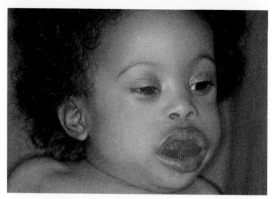

Fig. 176 Typical facies of Down syndrome.

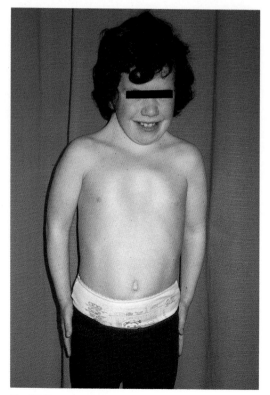

Fig. 177 Turner syndrome.

Sturge–Weber syndrome

Inheritance

Majority sporadic; occasionally autosomal dominant inheritance.

Clinical features

Facial port-wine stain, characteristically in the trigeminal distribution (Fig. 178), seizures, and sometimes mental retardation. A meningeal hemangioma is often present on the same side and may cause a contralateral hemiplegia, cerebral atrophy, cerebral calcification, and macrocephaly.

Klippel–Trenaunay–Weber syndrome

Inheritance

Sporadic occurrence.

Clinical features

Cutaneous hemangioma and asymmetric limb hypertrophy (Fig. 179). Associated arteriovenous fistulas are common, and lymphangiomatous anomalies sometimes occur.

Management

Surgery may be necessary when there is disproportionate limb growth or troublesome arteriovenous fistulas.

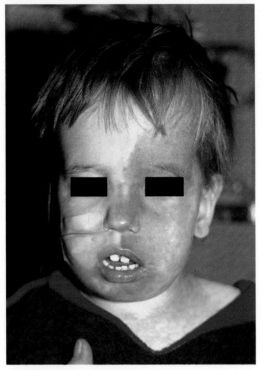

Fig. 178 Facial hemangioma in Sturge–Weber syndrome.

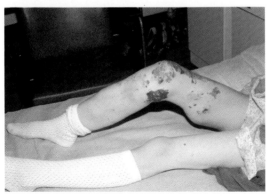

Fig. 179 Cutaneous hemangioma and limb hypertrophy in Klippel–Trenaunay–Weber syndrome.

Tuberose sclerosis

Synonym

Epiloia.

Inheritance

Autosomal dominant, but at least 80% are due to fresh mutation.

Clinical features

Severity and expression of the syndrome varies enormously, even within families. Usually epilepsy, mental deficiency, and some skin manifestations occur. All have granulomatous lesions (tubers) in the brain that become visible on CT scan by 7 or 8 years of age. Skin manifestations include the typical adenoma sebaceum (a papular rash on the cheeks) (Fig. 180), fibromas, shagreen patch, café-au-lait spots, and depigmented patches (Fig. 181). Visceral hamartomas and retinal lesions are common.

Waardenburg syndrome

Inheritance

Autosomal dominant.

Clinical features

White forelock (Fig. 182) or partial albinism and congenital deafness are usual. Sometimes, there is heterochromia of the iris and vitiligo of the skin (Fig. 183).

Management

Deafness is the most serious feature; usually bilateral and severe sensorineural deafness.

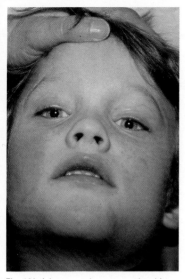

Fig. 180 Adenoma sebaceum on the chin.

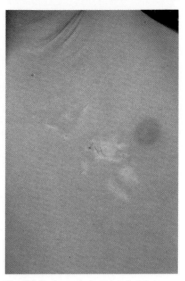

Fig. 181 Depigmented patches in tuberose sclerosis.

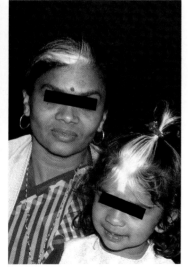

Fig. 182 White forelock of Waardenburg syndrome.

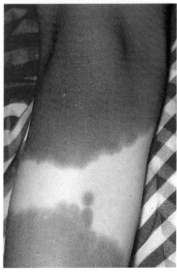

Fig. 183 Vitiligo.

Mucopolysaccharidoses

Inheritance

Autosomal recessive.

Etiology

Various specific enzyme deficiencies that result in accumulation of cytoplasmic mucopolysaccharides. Most common types are Hurler (type I), Hunter (type II), Morquio (type IV), and Sanfilippo (type VII) syndromes.

Clinical features

The infant appears normal at birth. Coarse facies (Fig. 184), growth retardation, mental retardation, skeletal abnormalities (Fig. 185), and hepatosplenomegaly gradually progress and become obvious within the first 2 years of life. Cloudy cornea is found in Hurler syndrome. In Morquio syndrome, there is severe skeletal deformity (Fig. 186) and growth retardation but normal intelligence.

Management

There is no cure, but bone marrow transplantation may be a useful form of treatment to halt the progression of the condition and may cause it to regress.

Short-limbed dwarfism

Incidence

Achondroplasia, the most common chondrodysplasia, occurs in about 1 in 10,000 live births.

Inheritance

Autosomal dominant, but the majority are fresh mutations.

Clinical features

Short stature, short limbs, and macrocephaly always occur (Fig. 187). Specific diagnosis is usually made on radiologic examination.

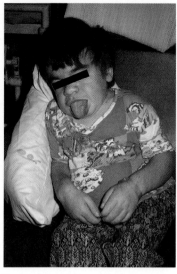

Fig. 184 Advanced mucopolysaccharidosis.

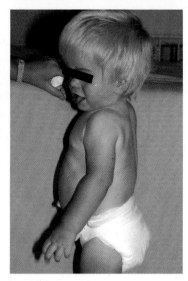

Fig. 185 Hurler syndrome.

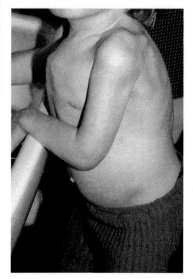

Fig. 186 Chest deformity in Morquio syndrome.

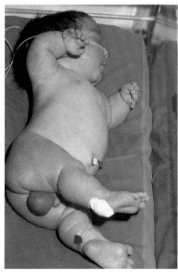

Fig. 187 Short-limbed dwarfism.

de Lange syndrome

Inheritance

Sporadic condition of unknown etiology.

Clinical features

Short stature, failure to thrive, and hirsutism (Fig. 188) are invariable. Bushy eyebrows (synophrys), long curling eyelashes, micrognathia, small nose with anteverted nostrils, and down-turned mouth (Fig. 189) give a characteristic facial appearance.

Course and prognosis

All are severely mentally retarded, and death usually occurs in early childhood.

Crouzon syndrome

Inheritance

Autosomal dominant with variable expression.

Clinical features

Cranial facial dysostosis with craniosynostosis of coronal, lambdoid, and sagittal sutures. Ocular proptosis because of shallow orbits and hypertelorism give a characteristic facial appearance (Fig. 190).

Management

Surgery to allow normal brain growth when craniosynostosis is severe or for cosmetic reasons.

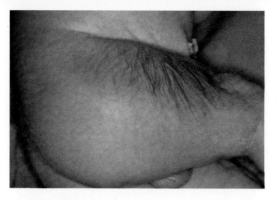

Fig. 188 Particularly hairy leg in a baby with de Lange syndrome.

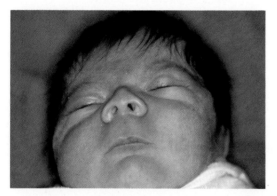

Fig. 189 Characteristic facial appearance in de Lange syndrome.

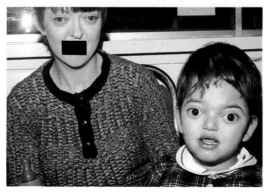

Fig. 190 Crouzon syndrome. (By courtesy of Dr. A. Kilby.)

Progeria

Extremely rare syndrome of unknown etiology.

Most cases are sporadic.

Premature and rapid aging with onset in infancy. Severe growth retardation, loss of subcutaneous fat, and generalized atherosclerosis (Fig. 191). Alopecia, hypoplastic nails, and flexion deformities sometimes occur.

There is normal brain development and intelligence. Life expectancy is severely shortened (average, 15 years), and death is usually due to myocardial infarction.

Russell–Silver syndrome

Uncommon.

Usually sporadic.

A syndrome of extreme growth retardation of prenatal onset, asymmetry of the limbs, and shortened incurved fifth finger. There is craniofacial dysostosis with small triangular facies and a small down-turned mouth (Fig. 192).

Gradual improvement in growth rate may occur in later childhood, but final adult height remains small.

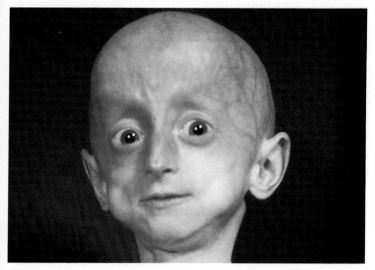

Fig. 191 Progeria.

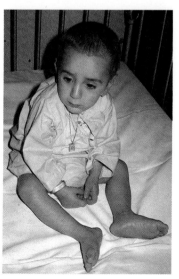

Fig. 192 Russell–Silver dwarfism.

Lesch–Nyhan syndrome

Inheritance   X-linked.

Etiology   Enzyme deficiency resulting in overproduction of uric acid; antenatal diagnosis now available for high-risk families.

Clinical features   Mental retardation, athetoid or choreiform movements, dysarthria, muscle weakness, brisk tendon reflexes, and extensor plantar responses. Characteristic self-mutilation (Fig. 193) due to uncontrollable aggressive impulses that appear to be unrelated to impaired sensation or hyperuricemia.

Management   Hyperuricemia can be controlled with allopurinol, but clinical course remains unchanged.

Lowe syndrome

Synonym   Oculocerebrorenal syndrome.

Inheritance   X-linked.

Clinical features   Mental retardation, hypotonia, joint hypermobility, hyperactivity, and growth retardation are common (Fig. 194). Cataracts and blindness usually occur. Renal tubular dysfunction and cryptorchidism are also found.

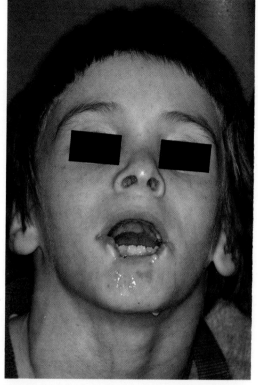

Fig. 193 Lesch–Nyhan syndrome showing effects of self-mutilation.

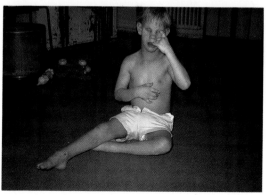

Fig. 194 A mentally handicapped blind child with Lowe syndrome.

Branchial arch syndrome

Synonym

Facioauriculovertebral syndrome.

Incidence

Relatively common. It is often associated with ocular or vertebral anomalies or epibulbar dermoids (Goldenhar syndrome).

Clinical features

Hypoplastic pinna with absent external auditory meatus (Fig. 195). Usually unilateral. Accessory preauricular tags are common. Unilateral hearing loss common, but speech is usually normal if hearing is normal on the other side. Facial hypoplasia and branchial cleft remnants in the anterolateral neck are common.

Management

Early assessment of hearing is important. Cosmetic surgery is usually desirable but not always satisfactory.

Ectodermal dysplasia

Incidence and inheritance

Rare; X-linked and autosomal dominant inheritance described.

Clinical features

Hypoplastic or absent nails and teeth (Fig. 196). Hair is usually fine and sparse. Abnormalities of sweat and sebaceous glands also occur in some varieties.

Nail–patella syndrome

Incidence

Uncommon.

Clinical features

Hyperplastic or absent nails and absent patellae (Fig. 197). Osteoarthritis of the knees develops in adult life.

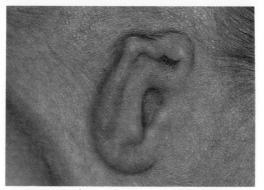

Fig. 195 Hypoplastic pinna with absent external auditory meatus.

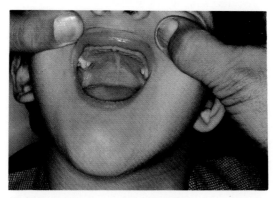

Fig. 196 Absent teeth in ectodermal dysplasia.

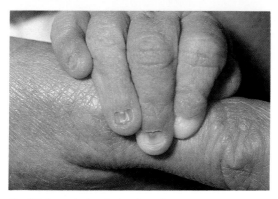

Fig. 197 Hyperplastic nails in nail–patella syndrome.

Menkes syndrome (Menkes kinky hair syndrome)

Incidence	Rare.
Inheritance	X-linked recessive.
Etiology	Probably a defect of copper-binding protein metalloprotein.
Clinical features	Characteristic sparse, twisted kinky hair (Figs. 198 and 199) that has partial breakages and twists on microscopic examination. There is profound progressive neurologic deterioration and failure to thrive from early infancy. Death is usual in the first few years.
Antenatal diagnosis	Excessive copper uptake in cultured amniotic cells has been demonstrated.

Cockayne syndrome

Incidence	Rare.
Inheritance	Autosomal recessive; antenatal diagnosis now possible.
Clinical features	Short stature with loss of subcutaneous fat from infancy. Dorsal kyphosis (Fig. 200), limitation of joint movement, gray sparse hair, and mental retardation are present. Retinal pigmentation and photosensitive skin are common.

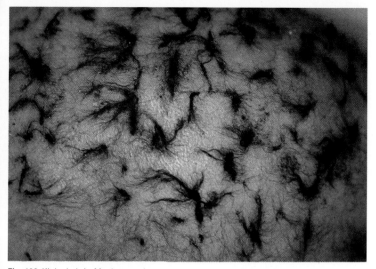

Fig. 198 Kinky hair in Menkes syndrome.

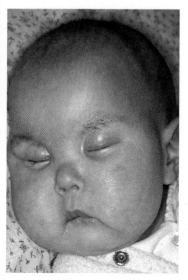

Fig. 199 Facies of Menkes syndrome showing puffy cheeks and kinky eyebrows.

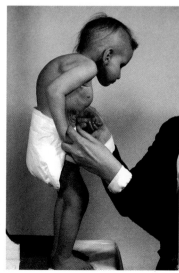

Fig. 200 Cockayne syndrome.

Vision

Myelination of the optic pathways is incomplete at term; early correction of congenital cataracts or severe ptosis is important for normal visual development. At birth, the child will fix for a short while on the mother's face and by 6–8 weeks follows objects in the direct line of vision. From 9 months, small graded white balls (Stycar test balls) can be used to test visual acuity. After 3 years of age, the child can usually match letters with graded letter cards (Fig. 201).

Hearing

The newborn infant will quiet with soothing noises and within a few weeks of birth reacts to loud noises by startling or crying. By 7–9 months of age, infants will turn their heads or move their eyes toward a sound stimulus such as a high-pitched rattle or bell at ear level (Fig. 202). Comprehension and imitation of normal speech indicate that severe hearing loss is unlikely.

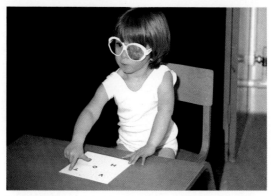

Fig. 201 Testing vision with graded letter cards in a 3-year-old child.

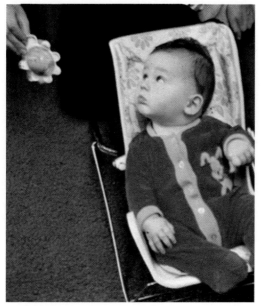

Fig. 202 Hearing test at 8 months of age.

Drawings

The pictures a child is asked to draw can provide useful clinical information. A child can be asked to "draw a man" and the parts of the body included in the picture are a good indication of the stage of development. Some pictures may indicate emotional problems that cannot otherwise be communicated to the clinician (Figs. 203–206). Sometimes the drawing may reveal an undiscovered clinical feature such as hemianopia in a child who only draws on one side of the paper.

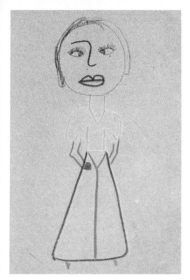

Fig. 203 Picture of a slim woman by a very obese girl.

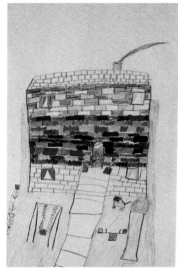

Fig. 204 "My house" by a child who lived in very poor accommodation.

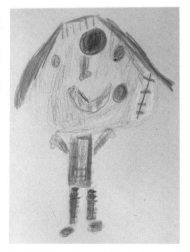

Fig. 205 "A man" by a child who had had a hernia operation. A lump and wound with stitches are clearly shown, although on different parts of the body from the operation.

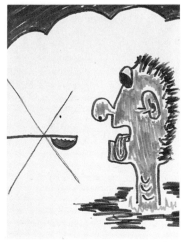

Fig. 206 "A man" by a child with food intolerance.

Admission to the hospital is distressing for all of us, but it is worse for children. A child younger than 5 years may not only be frightened by the illness and painful procedures such as intravenous infusions and blood tests but can be even more upset by separation from the family. It is very important that someone already known to the child should stay with them in the hospital; preferably this should be the mother or father (Fig. 207). They can often do some of the nursing care; they may feed and comfort a small child and can also do more complicated things such as tube feeding, watching intravenous infusions, and care of a tracheostomy. Parents, siblings, and other relatives on the ward often add to the work of the staff because they naturally expect to ask questions about tests and treatment they see. Even so, their presence helps all the staff to care for the ill child better and makes the hospital stay much less frightening. A controlled trial has shown that after-effects, such as nightmares, clinging, and a recurrence of enuresis, were less common in children whose mothers stayed with them in the hospital. A playgroup (Fig. 208) and a school are essential on a children's ward. Play (Fig. 209) allows the children to bear the strain of the admission and often reveals information about their physical and emotional problems. It is very important that a long illness should not interrupt school work.

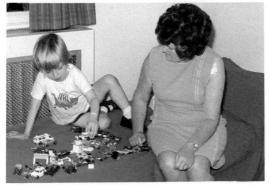

Fig. 207 Mother and child in the hospital.

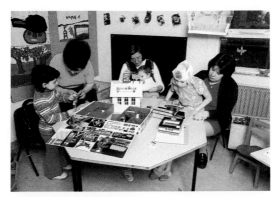

Fig. 208 Hospital playgroup with children and parents.

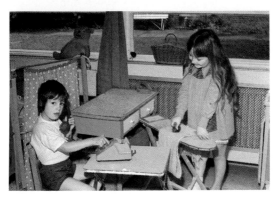

Fig. 209 Children at play during hospital admission.

Index